SELF-ASSESSMENT PICTURE TESTS IN VETERINARY MEDICINE

W0008357

DIAGNOSTIC IMAGING OF THE DOG AND CAT

Christopher R. Lamb
MA, VetMB, MRCVS
Diplomate, American College of Veterinary Radiology
Lecturer in Radiology
Department of Small Animal Medicine and Surgery
Royal Veterinary College
University of London
Hawkshead Lane
North Mymms
Hertfordshire
England

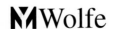

Copyright © 1994 Mosby–Year Book Europe Limited
Published in 1994 by Wolfe Publishing, an imprint of Mosby–Year Book
Europe Limited
Printed by BPCC Hazell Books Ltd, Aylesbury, England
ISBN 0 7234 1933 7

For full details of all Mosby–Year Book Europe Limited titles please write to
Mosby–Year Book Europe Limited, Lynton House, 7–12 Tavistock Square,
London WC1H 9LB, England.

A CIP catalogue record for this book is available from the British Library.

Library of Congress Cataloging-in-Publication Data has been applied for.

CONTENTS

Preface   vi

Questions   1
    Thorax   1
    Abdomen   28
    Musculoskeletal System   62
    Head and Neck   99

Answers   107
    Thorax   107
    Abdomen   127
    Musculoskeletal System   145
    Head and Neck   160

References   166

Index   172

PREFACE

This book represents another unit in the series *Self-Assessment Picture Tests in Veterinary Medicine,* a growing library of self-assessment material designed to promote continuing veterinary education. The self-assessment format is, as far as I am aware, new to veterinary radiology. Most existing veterinary radiology books offer variations on the text/atlas theme, usually providing comprehensive collections of images that cover the range of diseases and techniques encountered by the veterinary radiologist. In general, they represent excellent sources of technical, radiological and pathophysiological information but are less successful as means of developing interpretive skills.

This book aims to be different. It attempts to mimic the circumstances under which veterinarians practice radiology by presenting a series of diagnostic problems and the means to solve them. Admittedly, it represents an improved reality: the case presentations are straightforward (there are few red herrings), the radiographic and ultrasound images are selected for their high quality and all show relevant lesions. Real life is not always like that; however, my aim is to focus the reader's attention on the abnormalities in the images and their interpretation by eliminating distractions associated with the practical difficulties of the subject.

In another way this book attempts to be realistic because the majority of conditions depicted here are ones that practitioners commonly face. With a few exceptions, the radiographs were collected in a busy small animal practice over a 2-year period; most of the images are non-contrast 'survey' radiographs; no attempt has been made to cover the comprehensive range of diagnoses and techniques that a radiology text must if it is to be considered a valuable reference.

Most questions follow a brief clinical history; I expect that most readers will wish to use this rather than examine the radiographs unprompted. Many radiographs in this collection contain abnormalities that are readily apparent; correct interpretation will depend on a careful examination of the *location, number, size, shape, opacity, margination* and *secondary effects* of the abnormality, rather than simply finding it. When you make a correct diagnosis, congratulate yourself and move on. When you fail to recognise a lesion, misinterpret it, or forget a key differential, the answer should enable you to recognise that mistake and to avoid it in future. In some cases the answer will specifically state why your interpretation was erroneous. References are provided so that you may explore unfamiliar territory in more detail. It is hoped that you will emerge at the index with an increased knowledge of small-animal diseases and their diagnosis and, more importantly, with improved *interpretive skills*. This format should be useful for veterinary students, practitioners, and anyone studying for veterinary radiology certificates and diplomas.

I wish to thank my colleagues in the Department of Small Animal Medicine and Surgery at the Royal Veterinary College, North Mymms, and at the Institutionen för Klinisk Radiologi, Sveriges Lantbruksuniversitet, Uppsala, for examining the manuscript and making numerous good suggestions for improvements.

I have tried to avoid equivocal or controversial diagnoses; however, let me be the first to admit that I do not know it all. I would be grateful if any errors could be brought to my attention.

Christopher R. Lamb

DEDICATION

To Henry, Ros, Syd, Swarna, Margaret, Bryan,
Lynda, Elizabeth, Julie, Max, Liz and David – my family,
and to Larry, Jon, Phil and Mike – my teachers.

QUESTIONS

Thorax

1 Define *photographic density*.

2 When describing a radiograph, what is an *opacity*?

3 What four types of body tissue can be distinguished radiographically?

4 What tissue interfaces normally enable radiographic identification of:

(a) The heart?
(b) The left kidney?

5 A thoracic radiograph of a nervous dog is blurred. List potential reasons.

6 A thoracic radiograph of a panting Greyhound is blurred due to respiratory movement. List possible remedies.

7 A radiograph is obtained of a non-standard view of a large dog and is underexposed. An empirical decision is made to double the film density. How would you achieve this by adjusting:

(a) The mAs?
(b) The kVp?

8 A thoracic radiograph of a very fat Yorkshire terrier is obtained with the dog lying directly on the cassette on the table top. The resulting image is judged to be poor quality due to excessive scattered radiation, and a decision is made to repeat the procedure using a grid. The grid has a ratio of 6:1, 24 lines/cm, and a Bucky factor of 2. What adjustment to the mAs should be made when repeating the exposure?

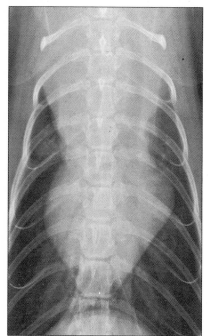

Figure 1

9 A 9-month-old male domestic short-hair cat had regurgitation intermittently for several days. The cat had been retching and the owner thought that something might be stuck in its throat. Physical examination was unremarkable. The cat was anaesthetised for an oral examination and radiography *(Figures 1* and *2).*

(a) What do the thoracic radiographs show?
(b) What is your differential diagnosis?

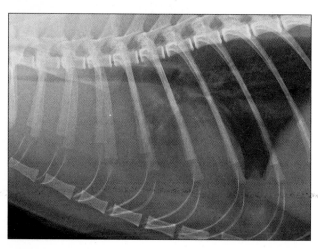

Figure 2

Figure 3

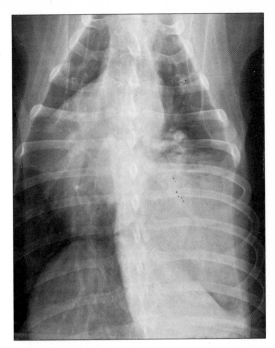

10 A 9-year old retriever had a cough for 6 weeks. The cough was intermittent, exacerbated by exercise and more marked at night. There had been some improvement following treatment using antibiotics; however, the cough recurred. Thoracic radiographs were obtained.

(a) Describe the lesion visible on this dorsoventral view (*Figure 3*).
(b) What is your differential diagnosis?

11 A ventrodorsal thoracic radiograph of a dog shows a mass in the area of the right middle lobe. Will this lesion be more visible on a left or right lateral recumbent view?

12 What quantitative radiographic criteria exist for normal feline heart size?

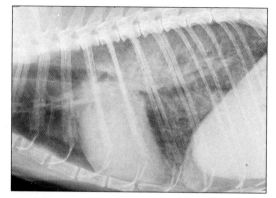

Figure 4

interstitial
pulmonary edema

13 A 13-year-old female domestic shorthair cat had reduced activity and inappetance. On physical examination the cat had pale mucous membranes, loud crackly breath sounds, audible third heart sound ('gallop murmur') and weak, rapid pulse. Thoracic radiographs were obtained (*Figure 4*).

(a) Describe the abnormalities.
(b) What is your diagnosis?

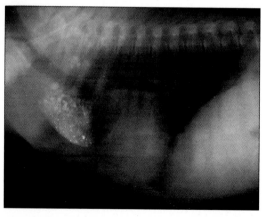

Figure 5

14 A 12-week-old male German shepherd puppy had persistent vomiting or regurgitation of food. It was not growing as fast as its littermates. Radiographs of the thorax were obtained.

(a) Describe the abnormality visible on this lateral view (*Figure 5*).
(b) What is your diagnosis?

4

15 List four clinical indications for an oesophagram.

16 Under what circumstances would you elect to use a water-soluble organic iodide contrast medium for an oesophagram?

Figure 6

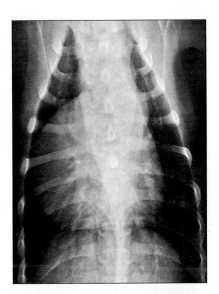

17 A 4-month-old male German shepherd dog had a loud systolic murmur, identified during a routine examination at vaccination. When prompted, the owner also reported that the dog's appetite was poor and the dog was thin. Thoracic radiographs were obtained (*Figures 6* and *7*).

(a) Describe the abnormalities.
(b) Can you make a specific diagnosis?

Figure 7

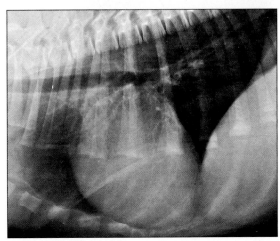

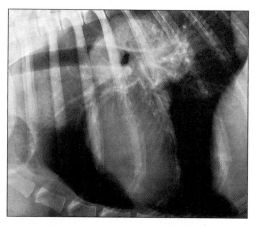

Figure 8

18 A 7-year-old female German shepherd-cross dog had inappetance, weight loss, polyuria and polydipsia. Haematology and serum chemistry values were normal. Thoracic radiographs were obtained as part of a general medical work-up.

(a) Describe the abnormalities on this lateral view (*Figure 8*).
(b) What is your diagnosis?

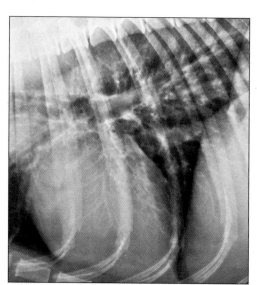

Figure 9

19 A 5-year-old male retriever had a chronic cough. Physical examination revealed a soft, apparently productive cough, which was intermittent at rest. Auscultation revealed increased breath sounds including high-pitched wheezing. There were no clinical signs of cardiac disease. Thoracic radiographs were obtained (*Figure 9*). What type of lung disease is present?

20 A 9-month-old male domestic shorthair cat had inappetance and abdominal distension. Physical examination also revealed hyperpnoea, muffled heart sounds and possible enlargement of mesenteric lymph nodes on palpation. Thoracic and abdominal radiographs were obtained (*Figures 10* and *11*).

(a) Describe the thoracic abnormalities.
(b) What is your differential diagnosis?

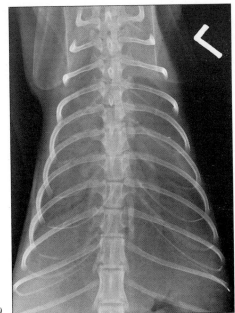

Figure 10

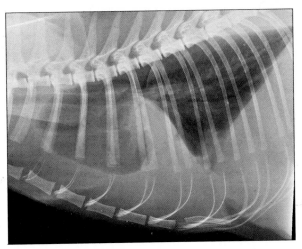

Figure 11

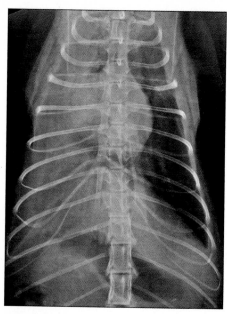

Figure 12

21 A 2-year-old neutered male domestic shorthair cat was hit by a car. When examined several hours later it was depressed, pale and dyspnoeic. Thoracic radiographs of the conscious cat were obtained (*Figures 12* and *13*).

(a) Describe the abnormalities.
(b) What is your diagnosis?
(c) What other tests might be used to confirm this diagnosis?

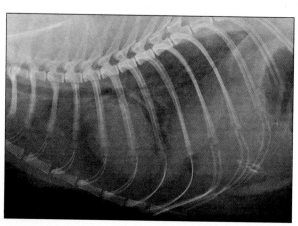

Figure 13

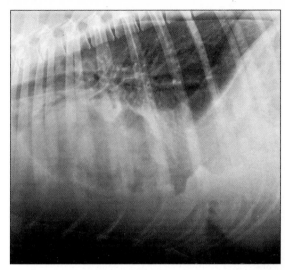

Figure 14

22 A 3-year-old male retriever had inappetance, depression and dyspnoea for several days. Physical examination showed increased inspiratory effort and pyrexia. The thorax was dull on percussion and the heart sounds were muffled on auscultation. Pleural fluid was suspected and blood-stained fluid was withdrawn by thoracocentesis on the left side. Thoracic radiographs were then obtained (*Figures 14* and *15*). Do the radiographs provide any clues to the aetiology of the pleural fluid in this case?

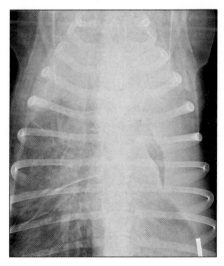

Figure 15

23 A 12-year-old neutered male domestic shorthair cat had lethargy, inappetance and weight loss. Physical examination revealed moderate dehydration and small, irregular kidneys; the cat's breath smelt like urine. A tentative diagnosis of kidney failure was made and blood samples were taken for haematology and serum chemistry determinations. Lateral thoracic (*Figure 16*) and abdominal (*Figure 17*) radiographs were also obtained.

(a) Describe the lesions.
(b) What is their significance?

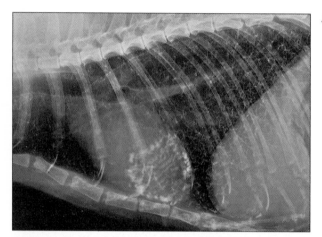

Figure 16

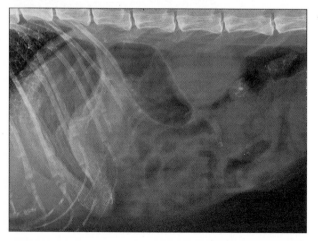

Figure 17

24 A healthy 2-year-old male Irish setter was admitted for routine castration. The dog was in lean body condition, but the heart sounds were judged to be muffled on pre-anaesthetic examination. Precautionary thoracic radiographs were obtained.

(a) Describe the lesions on this lateral view (*Figure 18*).
(b) What is your diagnosis?

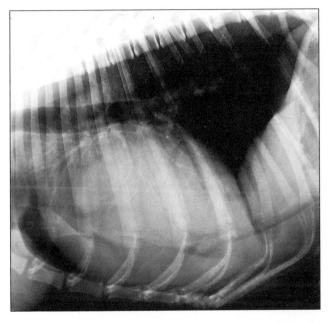

Figure 18

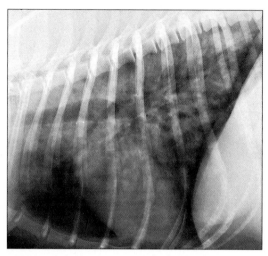

Figure 19

25 A 2-year-old male Jack Russell terrier had dyspnoea when collected from kennels by the owner, and then developed haemoptysis. The dog was presented to the vet weak, pale and distressed. No cough was observed. Thoracic radiographs were obtained (*Figures 19* and *20*).

(a) Describe the lesion.
(b) What is your differential diagnosis?

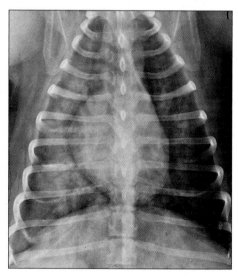

Figure 20

26 A 6-year-old female Dobermann had difficulty breathing, which became progressively worse over a 12-hour period. The dog seemed well the previous day and had enjoyed a long walk. Physical examination showed cyanosis, cool mucous membranes with slow capillary refill, rapid, weak pulse and loud, crackling respiratory sounds which prevented auscultation of the heart. Thoracic radiographs were obtained immediately without sedation (*Figures 21* and *22*).

(a) Describe the abnormalities.
(b) What is your differential diagnosis?

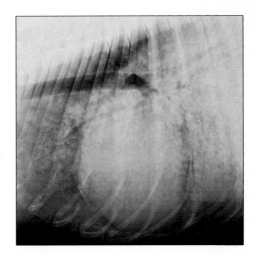

Figure 21

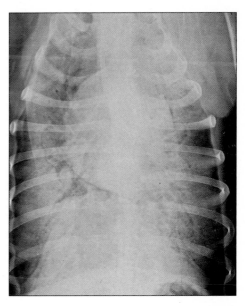

Figure 22

27 A 7-year-old neutered male Siamese cat was inappetant and appeared agitated; it had vomited once. Physical examination revealed a heart rate of 200 beats/min and a weak pulse. Increased breath sounds were identified on auscultation. Rectal temperature was 39 °C. Thoracic radiographs were obtained.

(a) Describe the abnormalities visible on this lateral view (*Figure 23*).
(b) What differential diagnoses would you consider?

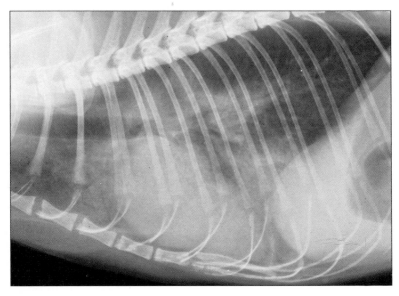

Figure 23

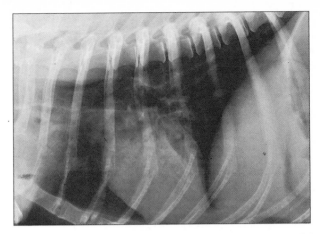

Figure 24

28 A 5-year-old male Dachshund was hit by a car. Physical examination showed paraplegia and dyspnoea. Thoracic radiographs were obtained without sedation (*Figures 24* and *25*).

(a) Describe the abnormalities seen.
(b) What is the lung lesion?

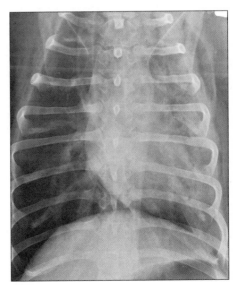

Figure 25

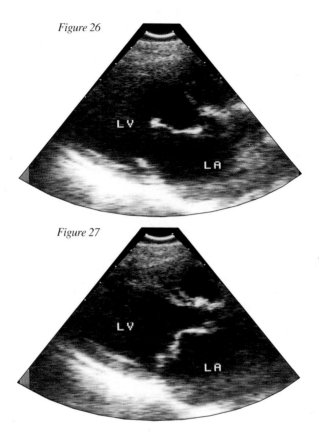

Figure 26

Figure 27

29 A 9-year-old male Cavalier King Charles spaniel had exercise intolerance and a cough for about 2 weeks. Physical examination revealed a rapid pulse, loud crackles in both dorsal lung fields and a systolic cardiac murmur, which was loudest on the left. Thoracic radiographs showed cardiomegaly and dorsal lung infiltrate compatible with oedema. Echocardiography was performed.

(a) What lesion is visible on these systolic (*Figure 26*) and diastolic (*Figure 27*) long-axis views of the left ventricle (LV) and left atrium (LA)?

(b) What additional abnormalities are indicated by the following echocardiographic measurements taken from other views?
- Aortic root dimension 17 mm.
- Left atrial dimension 33 mm.
- Left ventricular internal dimension in systole (LVS) 28 mm; in diastole (LVD) 48 mm.

30 A mature neutered male domestic shorthair cat was described by its owner as 'off colour' without any specific signs. On physical examination the cat had a rapid pulse and 'gallop' cardiac rhythm. Cardiomyopathy was suspected and thoracic radiographs were obtained (*Figures 28* and *29*). Do the radiographic findings support a diagnosis of cardiomyopathy?

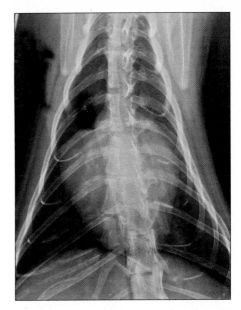

Figure 28

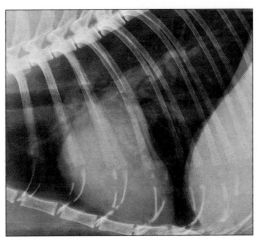

Figure 29

31 List the differential diagnoses for cranial mediastinal mass in the dog.

32 Thoracic radiographs are obtained of a dog with a known primary tumour, in order to look for evidence of metastasis. Several opacities are identified which are thought to be either small nodules or pulmonary vessels seen end-on. List three features of end-on pulmonary vessels that distinguish them from nodules.

33 Examine this lateral thoracic radiograph (*Figure 30*) of a 3-year-old female Dobermann.

(a) Describe the pulmonary pattern.
(b) What differential diagnoses would you consider?

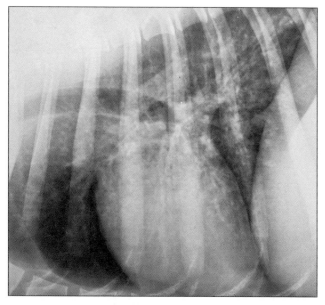

Figure 30

34 A 9-year-old neutered male German shepherd dog had a persistent low-grade cough, which the owner said was most noticeable in the evenings and sounded like the dog was clearing its throat. The dog was thin and vomited occasionally. Increased breath sounds were apparent on auscultation. Thoracic radiographs were obtained. Describe the abnormalities visible on this lateral view (*Figure 31*).

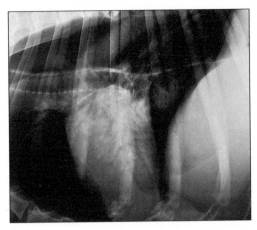

Figure 31

Figure 32

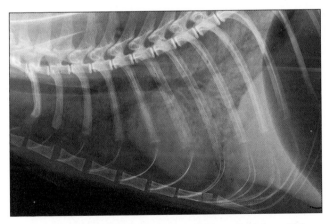

35 A 1-year-old male Persian cat was excitable and twitchy, which progressed over the course of a few days to an epileptiform fit. Physical examination revealed depression, blindness and hyperpnoea. Crackles were heard on auscultation of the thorax. Thoracic radiographs were obtained.

(a) Describe the lesion on this lateral view (*Figure 32*).
(b) How might this be related to the central nervous system signs?

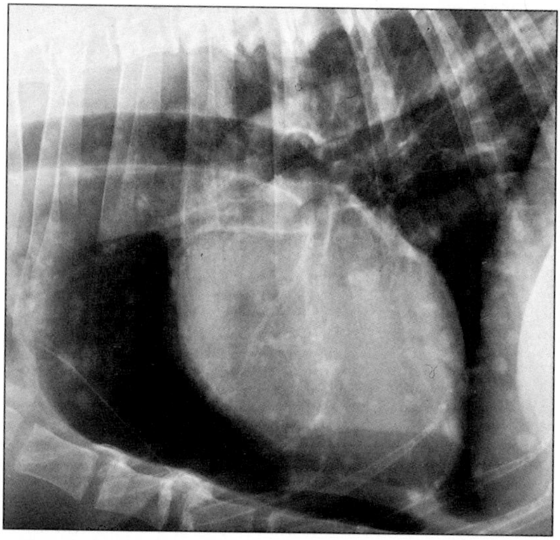

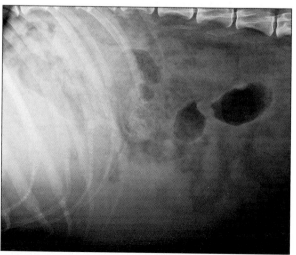

Figure 33

36 A 7-year-old male German shepherd dog collapsed at home. Physical examination revealed the dog to be thin, with pale mucous membranes, weak pulse, hyperpnoea and distended abdomen. Thoracic (*Figure 33*) and abdominal (*Figure 34*) radiographs were obtained.

(a) Describe the abnormalities.
(b) What is your diagnosis?

Figure 34

Figure 35

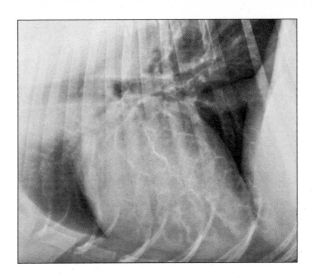

37 A 2-year-old cross-bred bitch had a chronic, productive cough that did not improve after administration of antibiotics or prednisone. Thoracic radiographs were obtained (*Figures 35* and *36*).

(a) Describe the abnormalities.
(b) What is your diagnosis?

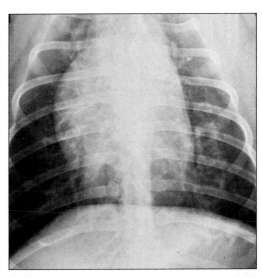

Figure 36

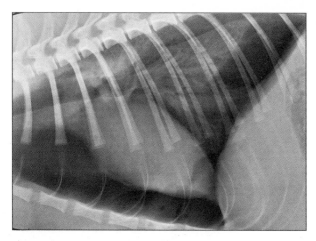

Figure 37

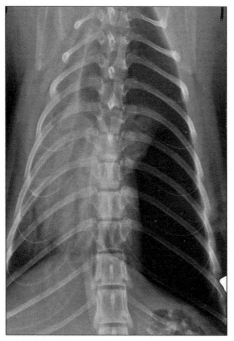

38 A 6-month-old male domestic shorthair cat had a wound on the left ventral aspect of its thoracic wall. The cause was unknown. The cat was hyperpnoeic and thoracic radiographs were obtained to identify any intrathoracic injury (*Figures 37* and *38*).

(a) Describe the abnormalities.
(b) What is your diagnosis?
(c) Is any treatment necessary?

Figure 38

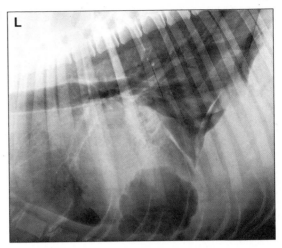

Figure 39

39 A young male stray cross-bred dog had been hit by a car and was brought by the police to the veterinary hospital for observation. The dog was bright but had evidence of pain on palpation of its trunk, bruises on its abdominal wall and hyperpnoea. The lung sounds were muffled on auscultation. Left (*Figure 39*) and right (*Figure 40*) lateral recumbent views were obtained.

(a) Describe your findings.
(b) What are your differential diagnoses?

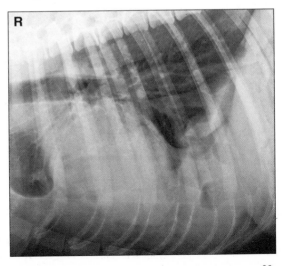

Figure 40

Figure 41

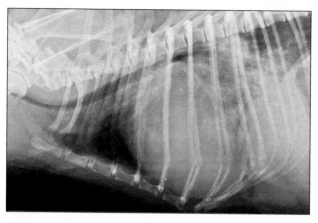

40 A 9-year-old neutered male Miniature Poodle had a chronic cough which was getting worse. The dog had, until recently, coughed only when excited but now coughed at rest, particularly at night. Thoracic radiographs were obtained.

(a) What abnormalities are present on this lateral view (*Figure 41*)?
(b) Are they related?

41 Study this lateral thoracic radiograph of a 7-year-old male German shepherd dog (*Figure 42*).

(a) What diagnostic procedure has been performed?
(b) What abnormality is visible?
(c) What is your differential diagnosis?

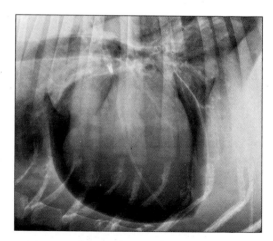

Figure 42

42 List the potential survey radiographic signs of thoracic mycosis in the dog.

43 The radiographic finding of calcification of the tracheobronchial lymph nodes is characteristic of which mycotic disease?

44 List the potential survey radiographic signs of *Dirofilaria immitis* infection ('heartworm disease') in the dog.

45 List differential diagnoses for pericardial fluid in:

(a) The dog.
(b) The cat.

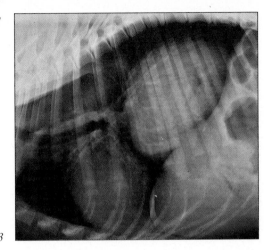

Figure 43

Figure 44

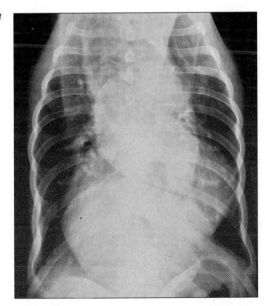

46 A 7-month-old male Shar-Pei had been intermittently regurgitating food or vomiting since purchase from a breeder. It was not gaining weight as fast as a littermate in the owners' care. Survey radiographs of the thorax and abdomen were obtained.

(a) Describe the thoracic abnormalities shown in *Figures 43* and *44*).
(b) What is your diagnosis?

Figure 45

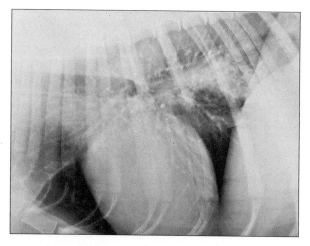

47 An 18-month-old male Labrador had a cough which had an acute onset and persisted for 3 weeks. The dog lived on a farm and was normally very active. Physical examination revealed no abnormalities. Thoracic radiographs were obtained (*Figures 45* and *46*).

(a) Describe the abnormality.
(b) What is your differential diagnosis?
(c) How might you confirm the diagnosis?

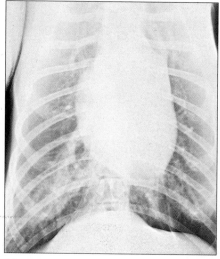

Figure 46

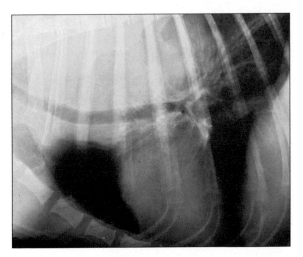

Figure 47

48 A 2-year-old male Irish setter had had difficulty swallowing for about 5 weeks. Solid food was regurgitated, although the dog could swallow fluid reasonably well. An oesophageal lesion was suspected and thoracic radiographs were obtained (*Figures 47* and *48*).

(a) Describe the abnormality.
(b) What is your differential diagnosis?

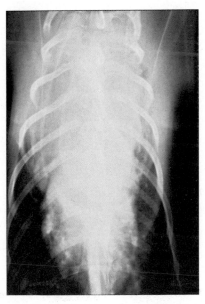

49 Give a list of differential diagnoses for cavitary lung lesions.

50 Give a list of differential diagnoses for the hyperlucent lung.

Figure 48

Abdomen

51 What quantitative radiographic criteria exist for normal liver size in the dog?

52 Give a differential diagnosis for generalised splenomegaly.

53 Give quantitative radiographic criteria for normal kidney length in:

(a) The dog.
(b) The cat.

54 A 9-year-old male Labrador retriever had weight loss, lethargy and reduced appetite. Physical examination revealed pale mucous membranes. No other abnormalities were apparent. Radiographs were obtained.

(a) Describe your findings on the lateral view of the abdomen (*Figure 49*).
(b) What further radiographic studies are indicated?

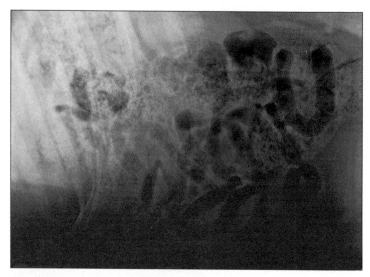

Figure 49

Figure 50

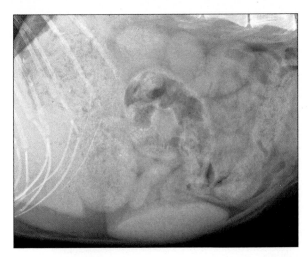

Figure 51

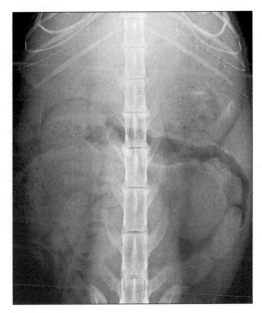

55 A 7-year-old female domestic shorthair cat had inappetance, reduced activity and weight loss. Physical examination revealed the cat to be thin with pale mucous membranes. The abdomen felt full but no masses were identified. Abdominal radiographs were obtained (*Figures 50* and *51*). What abnormality is apparent?

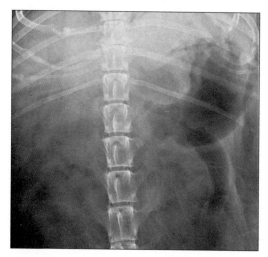

Figure 52

56 A 13-year-old female Cocker spaniel vomited for 2 days, then becoming depressed and anorectic. The dog showed signs of cranial abdominal pain on palpation. Abdominal radiographs were obtained. Describe the abnormality visible on this ventrodorsal view (*Figure 52*).

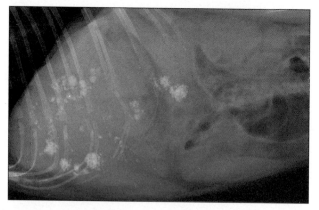

Figure 53

57 An 8-year-old female domestic shorthair cat had vomiting and lethargy for several days. Physical examination revealed the cat to be thin, with icterus, pyrexia and signs of pain on abdominal palpation. Abdominal radiographs were obtained (*Figure 53*).

(a) Describe the liver lesion.
(b) Do you think it is significant?

58 An 8-year-old male domestic shorthair cat had persistent vomiting for 2 days. The owner did not offer the cat food for 24 hours and the vomiting stopped; however, it recurred when food was offered again. On physical examination the cat was pyrexic and mildly dehydrated. Abdominal radiographs and a gastrointestinal contrast study were performed.

(a) Describe the abnormalities on the lateral survey radiograph (*Figure 54*) and the radiograph obtained 20 minutes after oral administration of barium suspension (*Figure 55*).
(b) Can you make a tentative diagnosis?

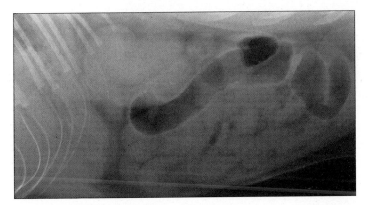

Figure 54

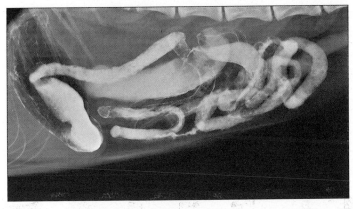

Figure 55

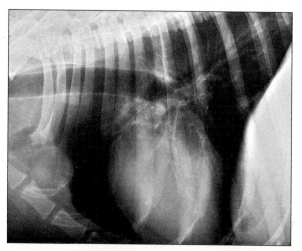

Figure 56

59 A 5-year-old female retriever had had vomiting and diarrhoea for about 1 month. The dog had a history of scavenging and had vomited plastic. When presented, the dog was listless, anorectic and had lost weight. Palpation revealed a cranioventral abdominal mass. Thoracic (*Figure 56*) and abdominal (*Figure 57*) radiographs were obtained.

(a) Describe the abnormalities on each radiograph.
(b) Are they related?

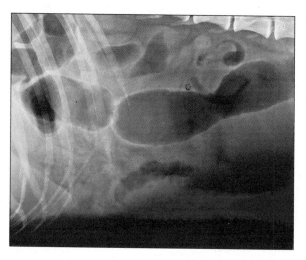

Figure 57

60 List differential diagnoses for a ventral mid-abdominal mass in a male dog.

61 A 5-year-old male English bull terrier was depressed, anorectic and had a distended abdomen. The owner thought that the dog had not defaecated for a week. The mucous membranes were a dull pink, capillary refill was slow, there was moderate dehydration and the abdomen was painful and full on palpation. Two lateral radiographs of the abdomen were obtained within a few minutes of each other (*Figures 58* and *59*). What is your diagnosis?

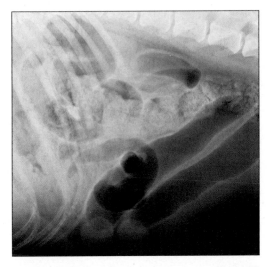

Figure 58

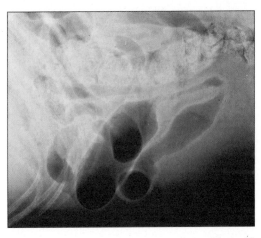

Figure 59

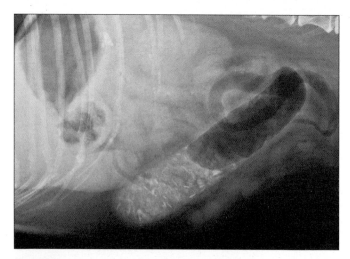

Figure 60

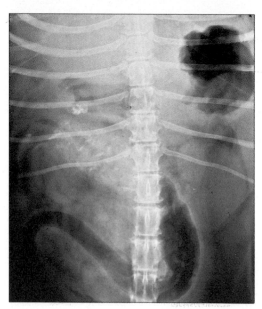

Figure 61

62 A 13-year-old neutered female Cairn terrier had intermittent vomiting, inappetance and weight loss for 2 months. The dog resented palpation of its abdomen but no other abnormalities were apparent. Abdominal radiographs were obtained (*Figures 60* and *61*).

(a) Describe the abnormality.
(b) What is your diagnosis?

63 A 20-day-old female domestic shorthair kitten displayed steadily progressive distension of the abdomen over a 3-day period. The kitten was eating normally and had no vomiting or diarrhoea. Rectal temperature was normal. Palpation revealed an enlarged viscus. Survey abdominal radiographs and a barium enema were performed.

(a) Describe the abnormalities on this ventrodorsal view after attempted barium enema (*Figure 62*).
(b) What is your diagnosis?\

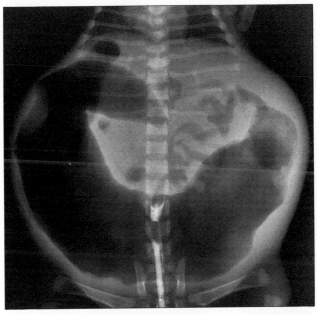

Figure 62

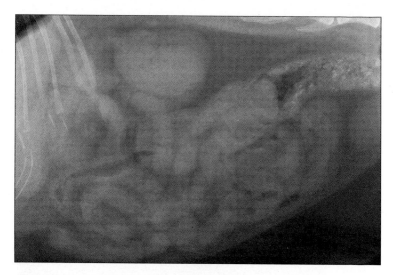

Figure 63

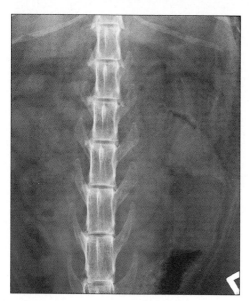

Figure 64

64 An 11-year-old female Siamese cat had inappetance for several days. A mid-abdominal structure was palpated but it was not clear whether it represented an abnormality or faeces. Abdominal radiographs (*Figures 63* and *64*) and an ultrasonograph (*Figure 65*) were obtained.

(a) What is your diagnosis?
(b) What is the prognosis?

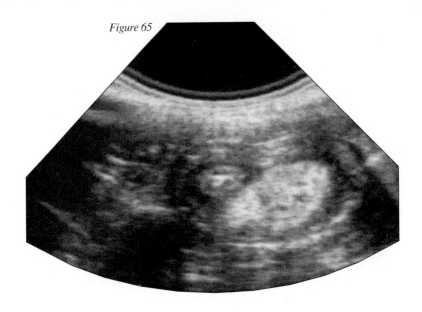

Figure 65

65 List differential diagnoses for bilaterally enlarged kidneys in the dog.

66 List differential diagnoses for asymmetrical kidney size in the cat.

67 What quantitative radiographic criteria exist for normal prostate size in the dog?

68 List differential diagnoses for calcified prostate lesions.

69 During investigation of a dog's enlarged prostate a retrograde urethrogram is performed, which shows marked reflux of contrast medium into the prostate. What is the diagnostic significance of this finding?

70 List differential diagnoses for a radiolucent filling defect on cystography.

71 List six clinical indications for intravenous urography.

72 A 13-year-old female collie-cross dog had intermittent vaginal bleeding which was not associated with oestrus. Vaginal examination revealed a pool of blood in the cranial vagina but no apparent lesion in the vaginal wall to account for it. The cervix was closed. Abdominal radiographs were within normal limits. A vaginourethrogram was obtained (*Figure 66*).

(a) Describe the lesion.
(b) What is your diagnosis?

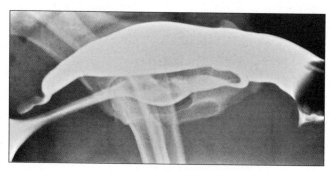

Figure 66

73 An 8-year-old male German shepherd dog had haematuria. Physical examination revealed prostatomegaly. The dog also appeared restricted in its range of movement when walking, although no definite lameness was identified. Radiographs of the caudal abdomen were obtained.

(a) Describe the abnormalities on this lateral view (*Figure 67*).
(b) What is your diagnosis?

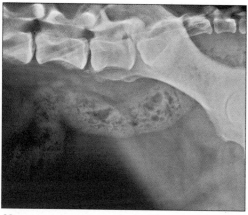

Figure 67

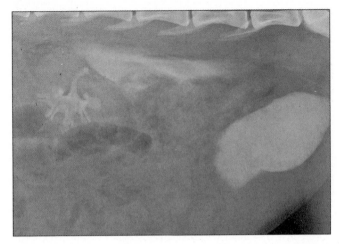

Figure 68

74 A 2-year-old female domestic shorthair cat was hit by a car and admitted for observation. The cat was depressed and had signs of abdominal pain and multiple skin wounds. After 24 hours in the hospital, haematuria and reduced urine output were noticed. Survey abdominal radiographs revealed loss of serosal detail compatible with peritoneal fluid. An intravenous urogram was performed.

(a) Describe the abnormalities visible in *Figures 68* and *69*.
(b) What is your diagnosis?

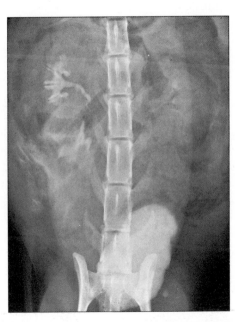

Figure 69

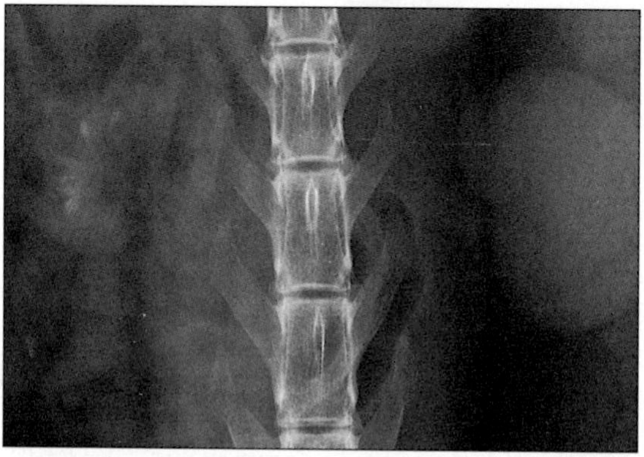

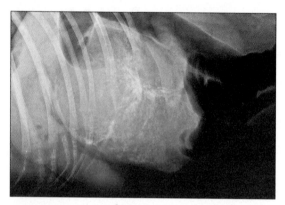

Figure 70

75 A 15-year-old neutered female Persian cat had depression, ataxia, proprioceptive deficits in the hind limbs and incontinence. Serum chemistry determinations included elevated urea (19.4 mmol/l), creatinine (211 µmol/l), hypergammaglobulinaemia, hypercalcaemia and hypophosphataemia. Abdominal radiographs were obtained.

(a) Describe the kidney lesions on this ventrodorsal view (*Figure 70*).
(b) What is your diagnosis?

Figure 71

76 A 9-year-old neutered male German shepherd dog had haematuria for 2 years. During this period the dog was castrated without any apparent effect on the haematuria. Physical examination revealed a large, hard, right-sided abdominal mass. Haematology and serum chemistry determinations showed neutrophilia, regenerative anaemia, and elevated liver enzymes and urea. Abdominal radiographs were obtained (*Figures 71* and *72*).

(a) Describe the lesion.
(b) Give two differential diagnoses.

40

Figure 72

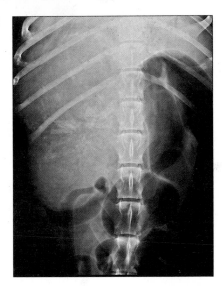

Figure 73

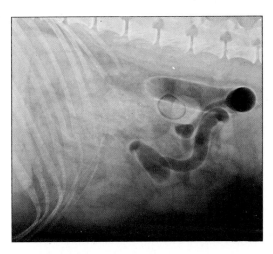

77 A 3-year-old female retriever was inactive, inappetant and vomited intermittently for 4 days. Physical examination showed mild dehydration, a full abdomen, a heart rate of 130 beats/min and a normal rectal temperature. Abdominal radiographs were obtained (*Figure 73*). What is your diagnosis? (Try to be specific.)

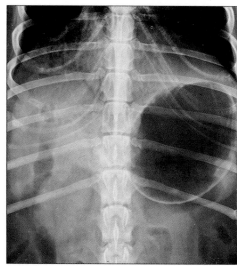

Figure 74

78 A 9-year-old male German shepherd dog had depression and weakness. Physical examination revealed mild icterus, pale mucous membranes, hyperpnoea, pyrexia and evidence of cranial abdominal pain. Abdominal radiographs were obtained (*Figures 74* and *75*).

(a) Describe the abnormalities.
(b) What is your diagnosis?

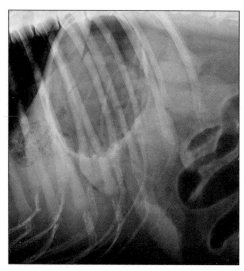

Figure 75

Figure 76

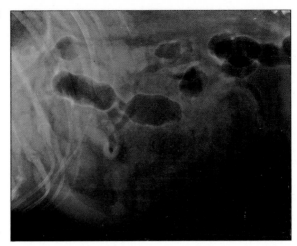

79 A 9-year-old neutered female cross-bred dog presented with chronic vomiting, inappetance, lethargy and weight loss. The dog resented abdominal palpation and the abdomen felt full but no definable mass was identified. An abdominal radiograph was obtained (*Figure 76*).

(a) What abnormalities are visible? (Compare with a normal abdomen, *Figure 77*.)
(b) What sort of disease could produce this appearance?

Figure 77

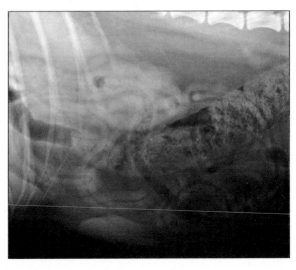

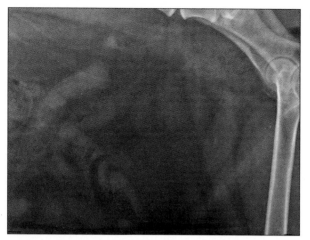

Figure 78

80 A 10-year-old neutered female cross-bred dog had a slight mucopurulent vaginal discharge and intermittent pyrexia. Previous treatment using antibiotics suspended these signs but they recurred as soon as the treatment was stopped. Radiographs (*Figure 78*) and an ultrasound scan of the caudal abdomen (*Figure 79*) were obtained.

(a) Describe the lesion.
(b) What is your differential diagnosis?

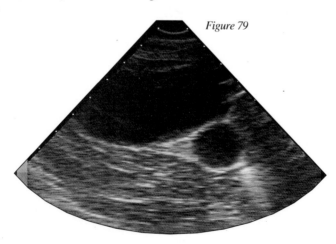

Figure 79

Figure 80

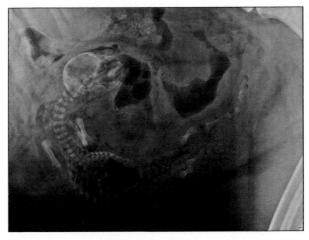

81 A stray female cross-bred dog of unknown age was found by the police and brought to the veterinary hospital. The dog was thin, appeared nervous but weak, and had a profuse green vaginal discharge. A large foetus was palpated. A survey lateral radiograph of the abdomen was obtained (*Figure 80*). Describe your findings.

Figure 81

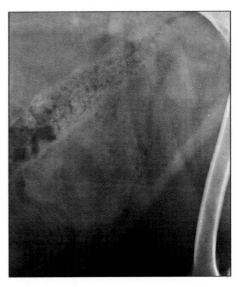

82 An overweight, 7-year-old male cross-bred dog had polyuria and polydipsia, haematuria and inappetance. Blood was taken for haematology and serum chemistry determinations, and radiographs of the abdomen were obtained.

(a) Describe the lesion on this lateral view (*Figure 81*).
(b) What is your diagnosis?

45

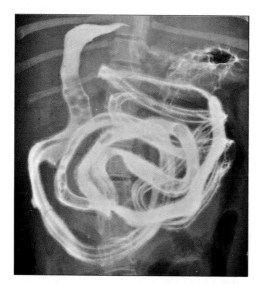

Figure 82

83 A 2-month-old cross-bred puppy had depression, vomiting and a small volume of diarrhoea. Abdominal palpation revealed no specific abnormality other than fullness. Survey abdominal radiographs showed no abnormality. An upper gastrointestinal contrast series was performed to rule out intussusception (*Figure 82*). What is your diagnosis?

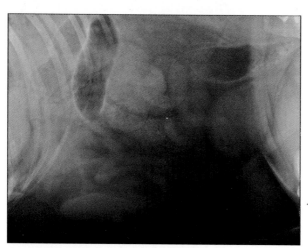

Figure 83

84 A 7-year-old male Corgi had polydipsia for 1 week. Physical examination revealed that the dog was overweight, had a thin coat, and one flabby testicle in the scrotum. Survey abdominal radiographs were obtained (*Figure 83*).

(a) What abnormality is present ?
(b) What is your differential diagnosis?

Figure 84

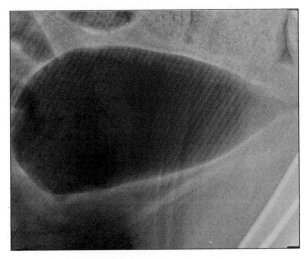

85 A 7-year-old female Cavalier King Charles spaniel had haematuria for 6 weeks. The urinary bladder was palpably thickened. A pneumocystogram and double contrast cystogram were obtained (*Figures 84* and *85*).

(a) Describe the lesions.
(b) What differential diagnoses would you consider?

Figure 85

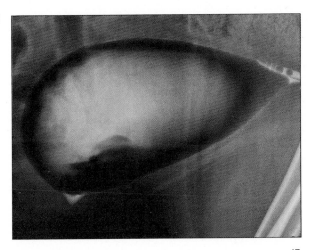

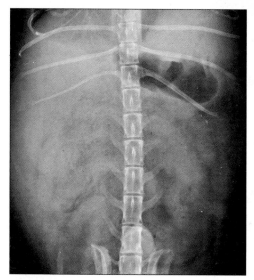

Figure 86

86 A 7-year-old male
Cavalier King Charles
spaniel had vomiting,
depression and cranial
abdominal pain for 3 days.
Survey abdominal radio-
graphs were obtained
followed by a gastro-
intestinal contrast series.

(a) Describe the
abnormalities on this
survey ventrodorsal view
(*Figure 86*) and on the
contrast study obtained 5
minutes after barium
sulphate administration
(*Figure 87*).
(b) What is your differential
diagnosis?

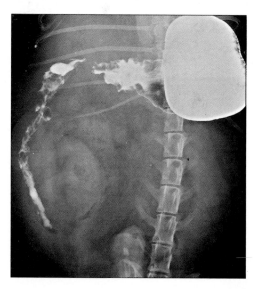

Figure 87

87 A 5-year-old female cross-bred dog vomited blood-stained ingesta and showed signs of pain on abdominal palpation. Abdominal radiographs were obtained to rule out a foreign body.

(a) Describe any abnormal findings visible on this lateral view (*Figure 88*).
(b) What would you do next?

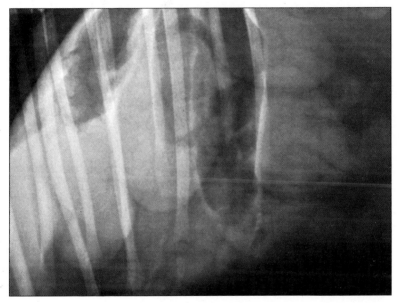

Figure 88

Figure 89

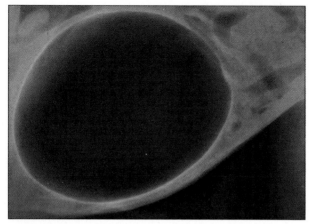

88 A 20-year-old neutered female domestic shorthair cat had haematuria and strained to urinate. Following treatment with antibiotics the clinical signs resolved for a few weeks and then recurred. The cat was unable to urinate when re-examined. Pneumocystography and retrograde urethrography were performed.

(a) Describe the abnormalities shown in *Figures 89* and *90*.
(b) What is your diagnosis?

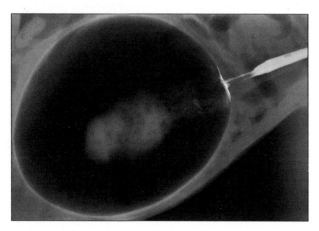

Figure 90

Figure 91

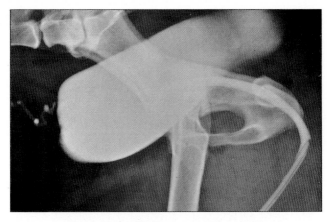

89 A 9-year-old male cross-bred dog strained to urinate and defaecate and had a perineal hernia. As part of the preoperative work-up, a retrograde urethrogram was performed (*Figure 91*).

(a) Describe the abnormalities.
(b) What is your diagnosis?

90 A 7-year-old male Labrador retriever had polydipsia and polyuria, vomiting, dehydration, hyperpnoea and a rapid weak pulse. Haematology, serum chemistry determinations, urinalysis and radiographs were obtained.

(a) Describe the abnormality visible on this detail of the abdominal radiograph (*Figure 92*).
(b) What is your differential diagnosis?

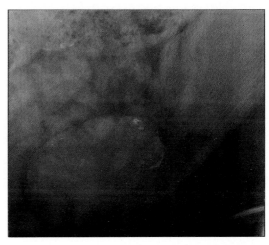

Figure 92

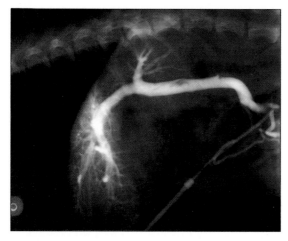

Figure 93

91 (a) How was the image in *Figure 93* obtained?
  (b) What does it show?

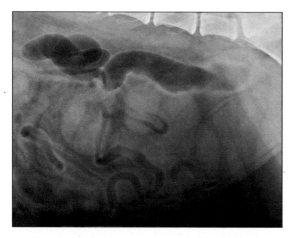

Figure 94

92 A 5-year-old female collie-cross bitch had depression, inappetance and polyuria/polydipsia and had vomited once. The dog resented abdominal palpation. A lateral abdominal radiograph was obtained (*Figure 94*).

(a) Describe the abnormality.
(b) What is your diagnosis?

Figure 95

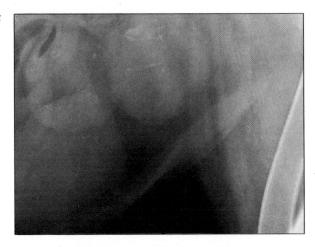

93 A 7-year-old, fat, male Rottweiler had haematuria. Blood dripped from the penis after urination. Abdominal radiographs were obtained prior to cystography.

(a) Describe the abnormalities visible on this lateral view (*Figure 95*).
(b) What is your diagnosis?

Figure 96

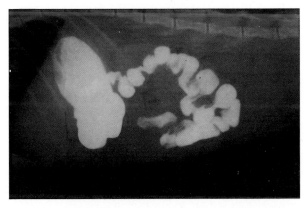

94 A 2-year-old male domestic shorthair cat had been vomiting for three days and was lethargic. Abdominal radiographs and gastrointestinal contrast study were obtained.

(a) Describe the abnormalities on this radiograph (*Figure 96*), obtained 30 minutes after oral administration of barium sulphate.
(b) What is your diagnosis?

95 A 10-year-old cross-bred bitch had intermittent vomiting, soft faeces and weight loss. A gastrointestinal contrast series was performed. What abnormality is visible in this detail of a ventrodorsal radiograph (*Figure 97*)?

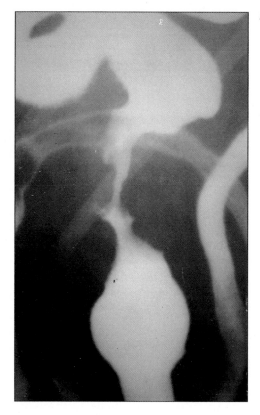

Figure 97

96 A 7-month-old Springer spaniel had clinical signs of hepatic insufficiency including elevated serum bile acid. An operative mesenteric portogram was performed (*Figure 98*), which confirmed portacaval shunt. A postoperative portogram was also obtained (*Figure 99*). (Please do not be confused by the stone in the intestine!)

(a) What has the surgeon done?
(b) What is the prognosis?

Figure 98

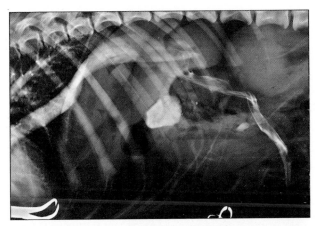

Figure 99

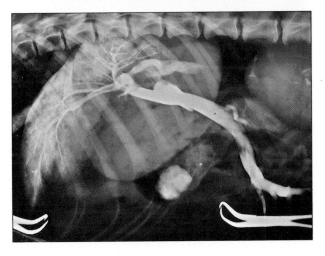

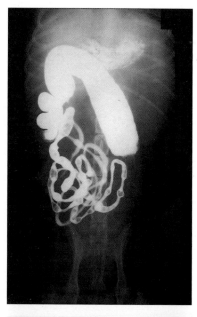

97 A 12-year-old neutered female Miniature Poodle had intermittent vomiting and diarrhoea for several weeks and became anorectic. The dog was thin and had pale mucous membranes. Survey radiographs were negative. A gastrointestinal contrast series was performed.

(a) What abnormality is visible on the ventrodorsal radiographs obtained 7 hours (*Figure 100*) and 22 hours (*Figure 101*) after oral administration of barium sulphate suspension?
(b) What is your diagnosis?

Figure 100

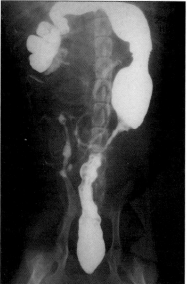

Figure 101

Figure 102

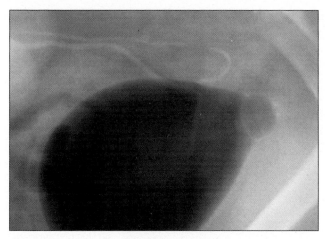

98 *Figure 102* is a radiograph of the caudal abdomen of a dog. How was this image obtained?

Figure 103

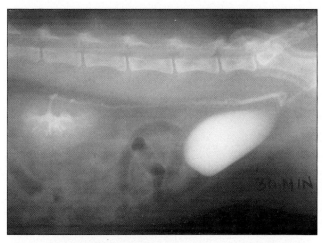

99 A 1-year-old female Siamese cat had chronic suppurative perivulval dermatitis associated with dribbling of urine. The cat used a litter tray and could void an apparently normal volume of urine. Intravenous urography was performed. Describe the abnormality visible on this lateral view, obtained 30 minutes after contrast medium injection (*Figure 103*).

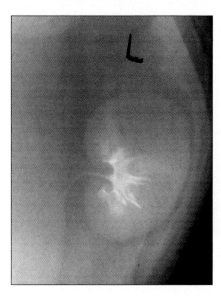

Figure 104

100 A 2-year-old female domestic shorthair cat had clinicopathological signs of renal insufficiency. An intravenous urogram was performed to evaluate the kidneys.

(a) Describe the lesions on this ventrodorsal view of the left kidney (*Figure 104*).
(b) What is your diagnosis?

101 A 7-year-old male Dobermann had ascites. As part of the diagnostic work-up, abdominal ultrasonography was performed. *Figure 105* shows part of the liver and spleen and peritoneal fluid.

(a) What abnormalities are present in addition to the fluid?
(b) What do they indicate?

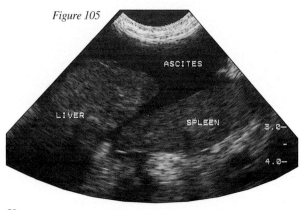

Figure 105

102 List differential diagnoses for a hypoechoic hepatic lesion.

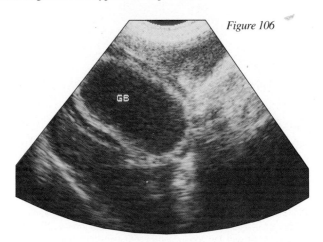

Figure 106

103 An 8-year-old female German shepherd dog had inappetance, icterus, abdominal distension and peritoneal fluid. Abdominal ultrasonography was performed. *Figure 106* shows the gallbladder (GB); the wall is diffusely thickened. Name two likely causes of this appearance.

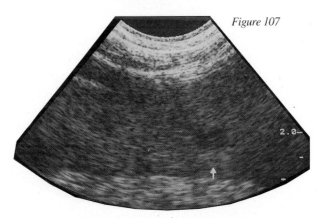

Figure 107

104 A middle-aged, formerly stray cat had lethargy, inappetance and weight loss. Haematology and serum chemistry determinations were unremarkable. Abdominal ultrasonography was performed.

(a) Describe the lesion indicated in this image of the spleen (*Figure 107*).
(b) What might it represent?

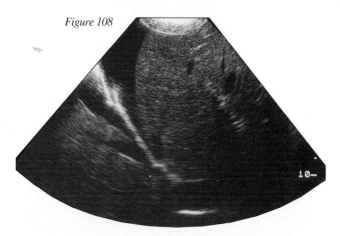

Figure 108

105 *Figure 108* shows a sagittal ultrasound scan of the liver and diaphragm of a dog with peritoneal fluid following trauma. What two artifacts are present that could contribute to a misdiagnosis of ruptured diaphragm?

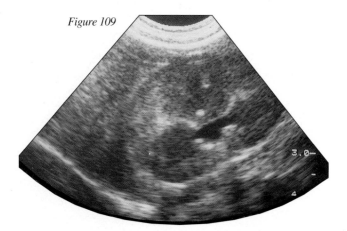

Figure 109

106 *Figure 109* is a dorsal plane ultrasound scan of the right kidney and adjacent liver of a cat.

(a) Name two abnormalities affecting the kidney.
(b) What is your differential diagnosis.

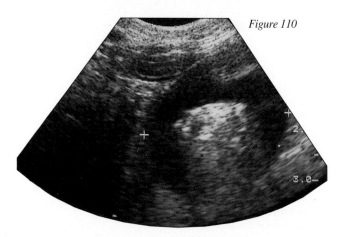

Figure 110

107 A 12-year-old female Siamese cat had inappetance, occasional vomiting and weight loss. Physical examination revealed a mobile abdominal mass. An ultrasound scan of the mass (between cursors) is shown in *Figure 110*. What is your diagnosis?

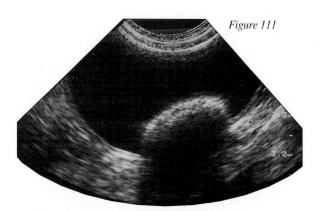

Figure 111

108 A 6-year-old female Miniature Schnauzer had vaginal discharge, polyuria and polydipsia. Ultrasonography was requested to rule out pyometra. During the examination a lesion of the bladder was discovered.

(a) Describe the lesion shown in *Figure 111*.
(b) What does it represent?

Musculoskeletal System

109 At what age do the following growth plates/centres of ossification fuse in the dog:

(a) Medial and lateral humeral condyles?
(b) Distal ulna?
(c) Anconeal process?
(d) Tibial tuberosity?

110 What single radiographic projection would be expected to provide the clearest view of the following lesions:

(a) Osteochondrosis of the tibiotarsal joint?
(b) Ununited anconeal process?
(c) Coxofemoral luxation?
(d) Zygomatic arch fracture?

111 A radiograph of a dog's paw is too dark for optimal viewing. List three possible reasons.

112 *Figure 112* is a lateral radiograph of the lumbar spine of an 8-month-old cat with clinical signs of back pain. Name two abnormalities.

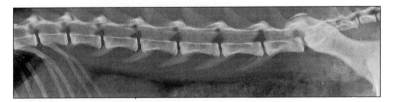

Figure 112

113 A 1-year-old male Bassett hound had been stiff and lethargic for several days. Physical examination revealed signs of pain on palpation of the hindlimbs and mild pyrexia. The dog was anaesthetised for detailed examination of the joints and radiography. Radiographs of the left femur (*Figure 113*) and pelvis (*Figure 114*) were obtained. What is your diagnosis?

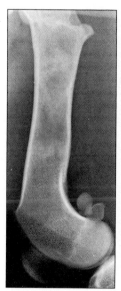

Figure 113

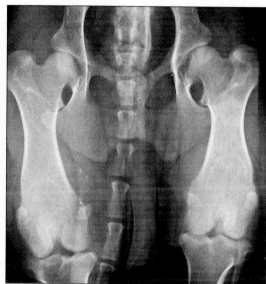

Figure 114

Figure 115

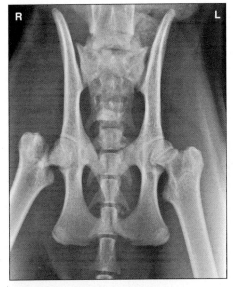

114 A 10-month-old male domestic shorthair cat was hit by a car, sustaining injuries to the hindlimbs. The cat was unwilling to stand, showed signs of pain on palpation of the pelvis, and crepitus was noticed on manipulation of the left hip joint. Radiographs of the pelvis were obtained (*Figure 115*). What is your diagnosis?

Figure 116

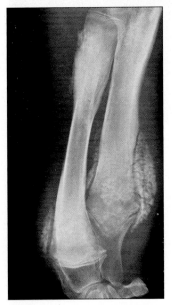

115 A 4-month-old female Great Dane was inappetant, depressed, pyrexic and had a cough. The dog developed mucopurulent discharges from the eyes and vulva 1 month later, and was barely able to stand due to painfully swollen limbs.

(a) Describe the lesion on this representative view of the left antebrachium (*Figure 116*).
(b) What is your diagnosis?

116 A 5-year-old male German shepherd dog had evidence of hindlimb weakness and was unwilling to exercise. The dog had difficulty climbing stairs. Physical examination revealed reduced hindlimb muscle mass and signs of pain on manipulation of the coxofemoral joints. A pelvic radiograph was obtained (*Figure 117*).

(a) Describe the abnormalities.
(b) What is your diagnosis?

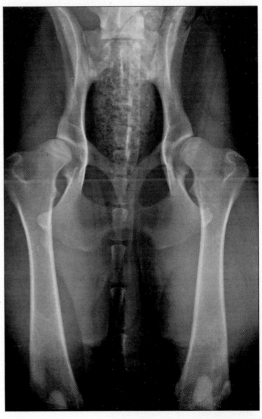

Figure 117

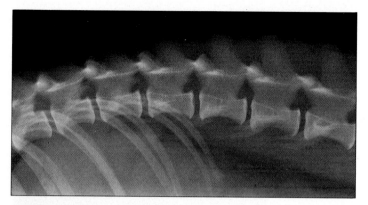

Figure 118

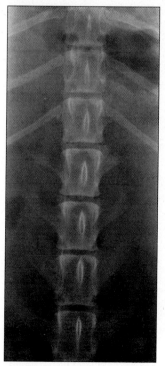

117 A 4-year-old male Toy Poodle showed signs of acute pain during play, then became withdrawn and inappetant. Physical examination elicited a pain response on palpation of the lumbar spine. There was good muscle tone in the hindlimbs and patellar reflexes were brisk. Survey radiographs of the lumbar spine were obtained (*Figures 118* and *119*).

(a) Describe the abnormalities.
(b) Which lesion do you think is responsible for the dog's clinical signs?

Figure 119

118 An unassuming 6-year-old male cross-bred dog had a fight with a stray dog at the park. It was lame and had a large laceration with extensive subcutaneous tissue damage around the left stifle. A fracture was suspected and survey radiographs were obtained. Describe the abnormalities on this lateral view (*Figure 120*).

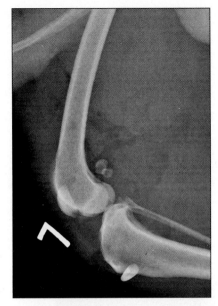

Figure 120

119 A 5-year-old male collie had acute left hindlimb lameness after a long walk. Pain and abnormal range of motion were apparent on examination of the left tarsus. Radiographs were obtained.

(a) What abnormality is apparent on the lateral view (shown in *Figure 121*)?
(b) What other views are indicated?

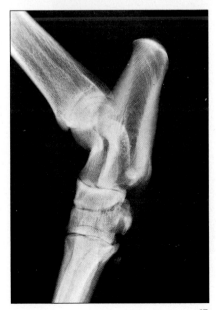

Figure 121

67

120 A heavy male Rottweiler becomes acutely lame during a run in the park. Based on the physical findings a ruptured cranial cruciate ligament is suspected. List the potential radiographic findings.

121 List diseases of long bones that principally affect the diaphysis.

122 List diseases of long bones that principally affect the metaphysis.

123 What four primary neoplasms are most likely to metastasise to bone?

124 A 4-month-old male Cavalier King Charles spaniel had acute non-weight-bearing lameness after jumping out of its owner's arms and falling to the ground. Swelling and crepitus on palpation of the left elbow indicated fracture. Radiographs were obtained (*Figures 122* and *123*). Describe this injury.

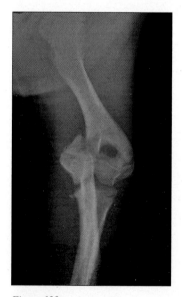

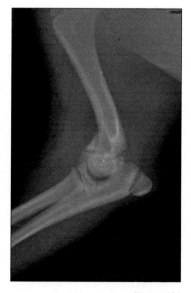

Figure 122

Figure 123

125 A 4-year-old male Great Dane had low-grade right stifle joint swelling and pain, which had been causing lameness for over 9 months. Radiographs were obtained after an acute exacerbation of lameness (*Figures 124* and *125*).

(a) Describe the abnormalities.
(b) What is your differential diagnosis?

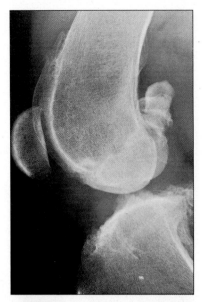

Figure 124

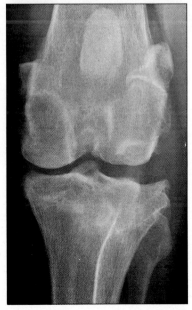

Figure 125

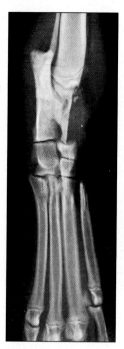

Figure 126

126 Study the dorsoplantar radiograph of the left hind paw of a young Greyhound shown in *Figure 126*. How did this injury occur?

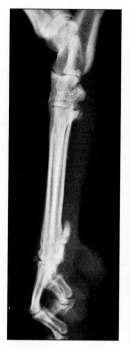

Figure 127

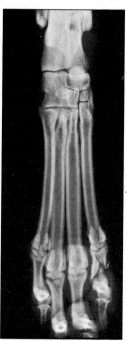

Figure 128

127 A 2-year-old neutered female Whippet became acutely lame after a fast run in the park. No trauma was observed. There was evidence of pain on palpation of the left hind paw. Radiographs were obtained (*Figures 127* and *128*). What is your diagnosis?

128 An 8-week-old female German shepherd dog was thin and had a cough and a painful right forepaw. Radiographs of both forepaws were obtained (*Figures 129* and *130*).

(a) Describe the abnormalities.
(b) What is your diagnosis?
(c) What treatment would you recommend?

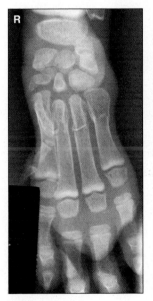

Figure 129

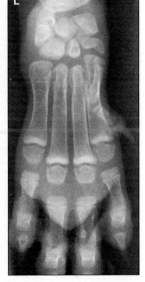

Figure 130

129 The right hindpaw of a 7-year-old male Rottweiler had been swollen for 2 weeks. The dog was inappetant, lame and pyrexic. Radiographs were obtained (*Figures 131* and *132*).

(a) Describe the abnormalities.
(b) What differential diagnoses would you consider?

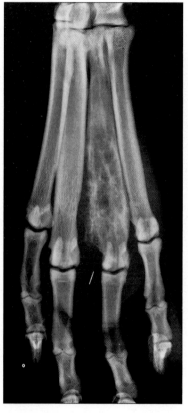

Figure 131

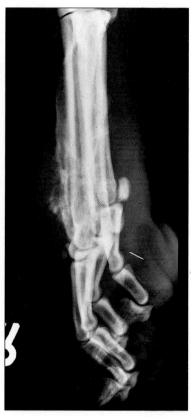

Figure 132

130 (a) How was the radiograph shown in *Figure 133* obtained?
(b) What abnormality is present?

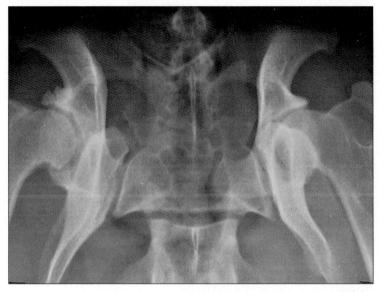

Figure 133

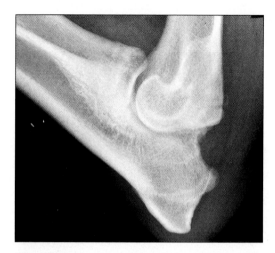

Figure 134

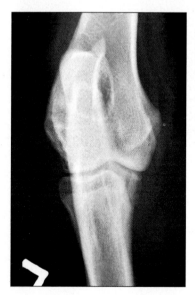

Figure 135

131 A 9-month-old female Rottweiler had a low-grade forelimb lameness for about 4 months. Palpation revealed swelling of the left elbow and signs of resentment when the joint was passively flexed or extended. Radiographs were obtained (*Figures 134* and *135*).

(a) Name two abnormalities.
(b) What is your diagnosis?

Figure 136

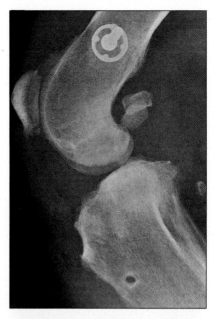

132 A 3-year-old male Rottweiler had persistent lameness, stifle pain and swelling several weeks after surgical repair of a cranial cruciate ligament rupture using a synthetic braided ligament prosthesis. Survey radiographs were obtained (*Figures 136* and *137*).

(a) Describe the abnormalities.
(b) What is your diagnosis?
(c) How might you confirm this?

133 List differential diagnoses for calcified lesions associated with joints.

134 You are presented with a dog for myelography. A thoracolumbar disc prolapse is suspected. Name any advantages of making the contrast medium injection at the level of the cisterna magna, and any advantages of using a lumbar injection site.

135 List the clinical indications for myelography.

136 Name the three categories of myelographic abnormality that are based on the location of the lesion.

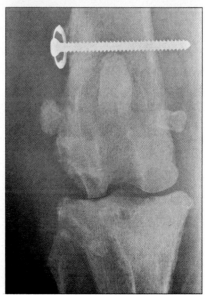

Figure 137

137 Name three potential causes of filling defects in the subarachnoid space on myelography (include anatomical, pathological or artefactual causes).

138 A 9-year-old male Dobermann had progressive difficulty rising and was ataxic. A cervical lesion was suspected and a myelogram performed. Radiographs were obtained with the cervical spine in a neutral position (*Figure 138*) and with traction applied to stretch the neck (*Figure 139*).

(a) Describe the myelographic lesion.
(b) How does its appearance change when traction is applied and what does this indicate?

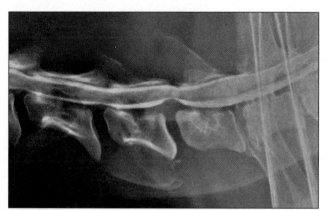

Figure 138

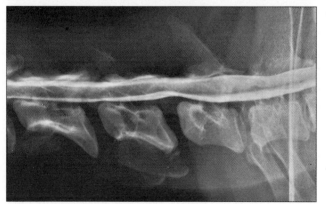

Figure 139

139 A 14-year-old neutered female domestic shorthair cat had an abdominal mass. Thoracic radiographs were obtained to rule out metastasis (*Figure 140*).

(a) What unexpected abnormality is present? (A radiograph of a normal cat is provided in *Figure 141* for comparison).
(b) What does it indicate?

Figure 140

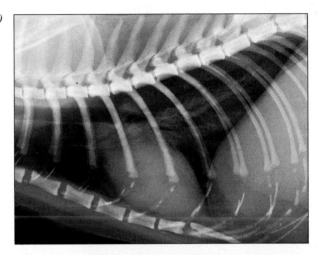

Figure 141

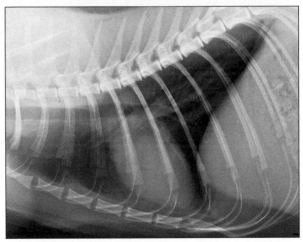

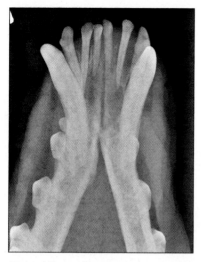

Figure 142

140 A 4-year-old male cross-bred dog had loose mandibular incisors and a firm, red gingival swelling. An intraoral ventrodorsal radiograph was obtained (*Figure 142*).

(a) Describe the lesion.
(b) What are your differential diagnoses?

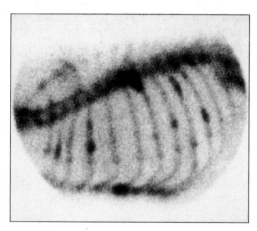

Figure 143

141 A 9-year-old male Schnauzer had dysuria and an enlarged prostate. Bone scintigraphy of the whole body was performed. A lateral view of the thorax is shown in *Figure 143*.

(a) How is this scan performed?
(b) What abnormalities are present?

142 A 1-year-old neutered male domestic shorthair cat had evidence of pain and swelling around the right hip. No other abnormalities were identified. Radiographs of the pelvis were obtained (*Figure 144*).

(a) What is your diagnosis?
(b) Is this an acute injury?

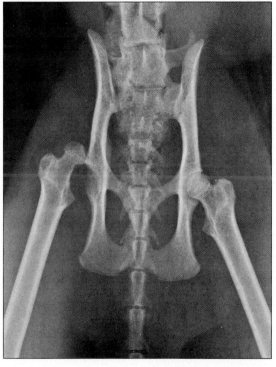

Figure 144

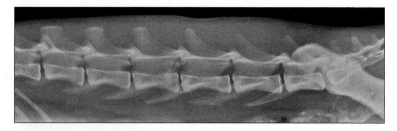

Figure 145

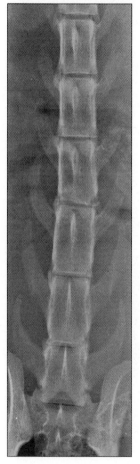

143 A stray female domestic shorthair cat (approximately 1 year old) was found on the side of the road unable to walk. Physical examination revealed paraplegia referable to a lower motor neurone lesion. Pain on palpation of the lumbar spine also indicated a lesion in that area. Radiographs of the lumbar spine were obtained (*Figures 145* and *146*).

(a) Describe the abnormalities.
(b) What is your diagnosis?

Figure 146

144 A 10-year-old female Old English sheepdog had chronic lameness associated with stifle arthrosis and hip dysplasia. The dog developed acute lameness of the forelimb and a hot, painful swelling of the carpus. Radiographs of the carpus were obtained (*Figures 147* and *148*).

(a) Describe the lesion.
(b) What is your diagnosis?

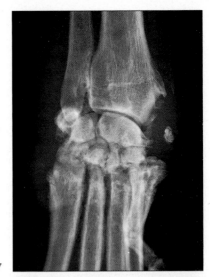

Figure 147

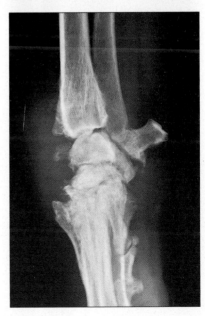

Figure 148

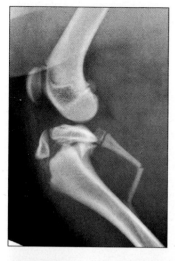

Figure 149

145 A 7-month-old West Highland White terrier had acute non-weight-bearing lameness after being trodden on by its owner. Pain, swelling and instability were evident on palpation of the left stifle. Radiographs were obtained. Classify the fractures visible in the lateral view in *Figure 149*.

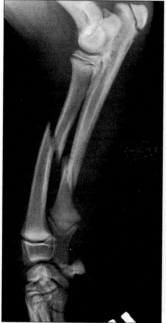

Figure 150

82

Figure 151

146 A 5-month-old male Cavalier King Charles spaniel trapped its right forelimb in a door and had acute non-weight-bearing lameness. Swelling and crepitus were apparent on palpation of the right antebrachium. Based on the results of the initial radiograph (*Figure 150*) the limb was supported in a padded splint and re-examined after 2, 4 and 9 weeks (*Figure 151*).

(a) Describe the fractures visible in *Figure 150*.
(b) What complication has occurred in *Figure 151*?

147 A 1-year-old female German shepherd dog was lame and had a painful, firm swelling over the right hip. Radiographs of the pelvis were obtained (*Figure 152*).

(a) Describe the lesion.
(b) What is your diagnosis?

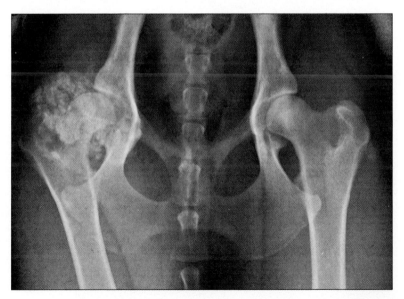

Figure 152

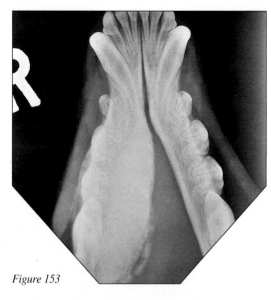

Figure 153

148 A 9-month-old male West Highland White terrier had diarrhoea, depression and a swollen jaw. The dog was pyrexic and had a hard swelling of the ventral aspect of the right mandibular ramus. Radiographs of the mandible were obtained (*Figures 153* and *154*).

(a) Describe the lesion.
(b) What is your diagnosis?

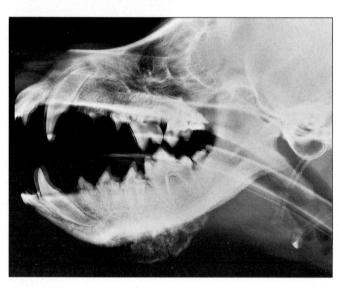

Figure 154

149 A 12-year-old neutered female domestic shorthair cat had acute pain and swelling of the left distal tibia. The owner thought that the cat had injured itself jumping off a chair. Radiographs of the affected area were obtained. How would you repair the fracture shown in *Figure 155*?

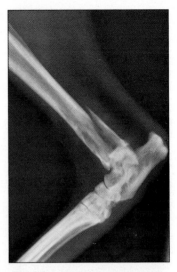

Figure 155

150 A 12-year-old female Whippet had been lame in its right hindlimb for 2 weeks. Physical examination revealed low body weight, painful swelling over the right femur and a 4-cm diameter hard mass in the left caudal mammary gland. Radiographs of the thorax were within normal limits.

(a) Describe the femoral lesion (*Figure 156*).
(b) What is your differential diagnosis?

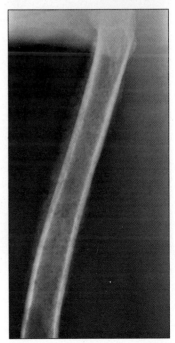

Figure 156

151 A 4-year-old female Boxer under treatment for ulcerative colitis developed lameness associated with a painful swelling of the left elbow. Pitting oedema was present distal to the elbow. A radiograph of the affected area was obtained (*Figure 157*).

(a) Describe the lesion.
(b) Is this joint disease or bone disease?

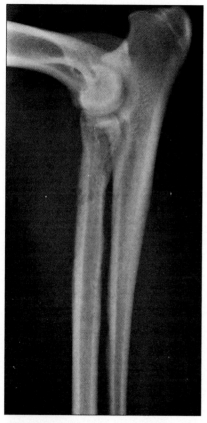

Figure 157

152 An 8-month-old female Boxer puppy had right hindlimb lameness for 1 week. Physical examination revealed a hard swelling proximal to the stifle. Radiographs were obtained (*Figures 158* and *159*).

(a) Describe the lesion.
(b) What is your diagnosis? (Be as specific as possible.)

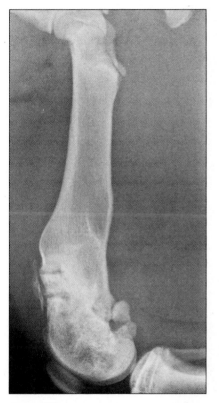

Figure 158

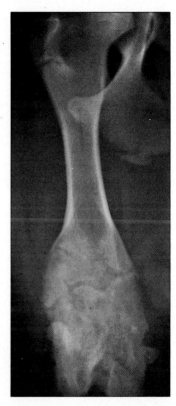

Figure 159

153 A 9-month-old male Border collie had persistent right forelimb lameness. Rest produced a minor, unsustained improvement. No lesions were apparent in the distal limb, but the dog appeared to resent manipulation of its shoulder. Survey radiographs (*Figures 160* and *161*) and positive contrast arthrograms (*Figures 162* and *163*) of both shoulders were obtained.

(a) What is your diagnosis?
(b) What arthrographic finding might indicate why the dog is lame on the right?

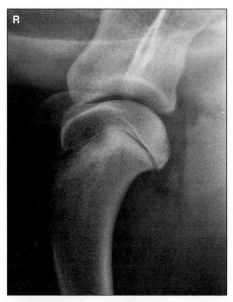

Figure 160

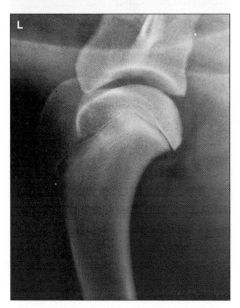

Figure 161

Figure 162

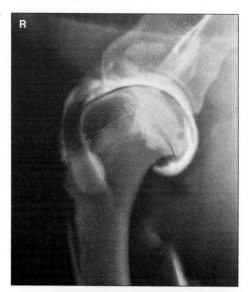

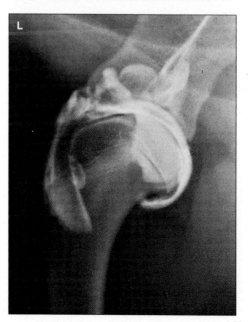

Figure 163

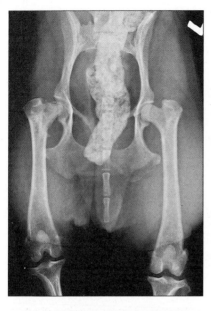

154 A 1-year-old female Yorkshire terrier had right hindlimb lameness. A radiograph of the pelvis was obtained (*Figure 164*).

(a) Describe the lesions.
(b) What is your diagnosis?

Figure 164

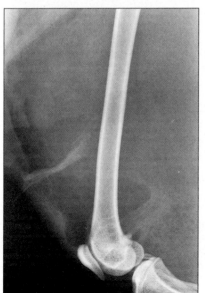

155 A 1-year-old male domestic shorthair cat had a laceration on the medial aspect of its right stifle, the cause of which was unknown. Palpation revealed swelling and crepitus due to subcutaneous emphysema. An angular, hard structure was palpated caudolateral to the stifle. Radiographs were obtained to rule out fracture (*Figure 165*). What is your diagnosis?

Figure 165

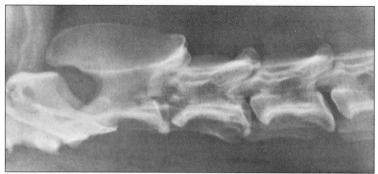

Figure 166

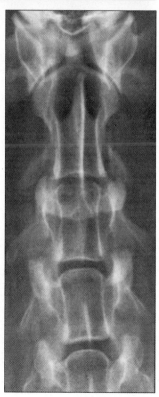

156 A 12-year-old neutered female retriever-cross dog had signs of neck pain, stiffness and left forelimb lameness for 6 weeks, which the owner believed to be getting worse. The dog was inappetant and thin. No neurological deficits were identified at physical examination. Survey radiographs of the cervical spine were obtained (*Figures 166* and *167*).

(a) Describe the lesion.
(b) What is your diagnosis?

Figure 167

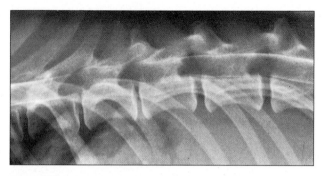

Figure 168

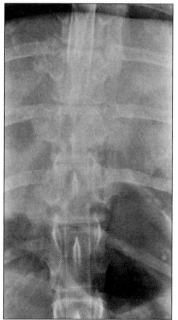

157 A 6-year-old male cross-bred dog was inactive and had bouts of shivering for a few days. It then became acutely paraplegic. Patellar reflexes were slightly exaggerated, the dog had no hindlimb pain sensation and was unable to urinate. A myelogram (*Figures 168* and *169*) was obtained.

(a) Describe the myelographic lesion.
(b) What is your diagnosis?

Figure 169

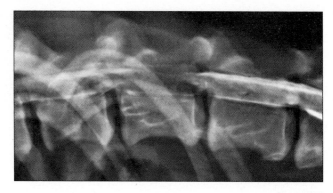

Figure 170

158 The owner of a 6-year-old male Boxer dog noticed that it scuffed its hindpaws when walking. This persisted for about a week. Physical examination revealed marked hindlimb ataxia, poor proprioception and bilateral crossed extensor reflexes. The dog showed signs of pain on palpation of the lumbar spine. Survey radiographs showed no abnormality. A myelogram was obtained (*Figures 170* and *171*).

(a) Describe the myelographic lesion.
(b) What differential diagnoses would you consider?

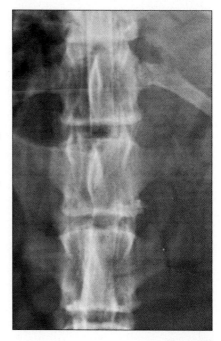

Figure 171

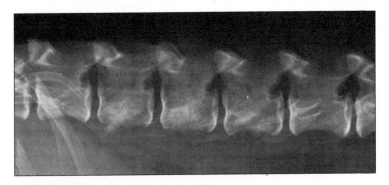

Figure 172

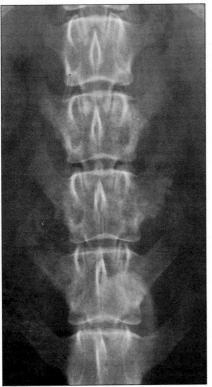

159 A 10-year-old male Corgi was progressively ataxic in the hindlimbs for 2 weeks and was then presented with acute paraplegia and signs of back pain. There was no history of trauma or previous illness. Radiographs of the lumbar spine were obtained (*Figures 172* and *173*).

(a) Describe the lesion.
(b) What is your differential diagnosis?

Figure 173

160 A 12-year-old Dalmatian had a gradual onset of hindlimb
weakness and intermittent signs of pain when sitting or rising.
Radiographs of the lumbosacral joint were obtained (*Figures 174*
and *175*). What is your diagnosis?

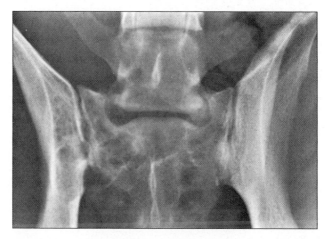

Figure 174

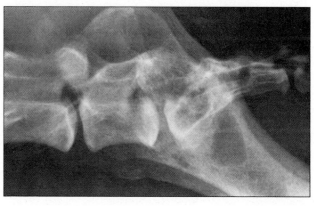

Figure 175

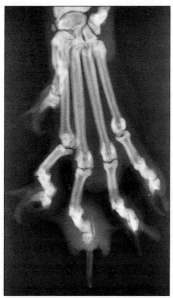

Figure 176

161 An 11-year-old domestic shorthair cat had a cough for about 2 weeks and a swollen toe. Physical examination revealed a very painful, reddened and swollen third toe on the right forepaw. Radiographs of the paw (*Figure 176*) and thorax (*Figures 177* and *178*) were obtained.

(a) Describe the lesions.
(b) What is your diagnosis?

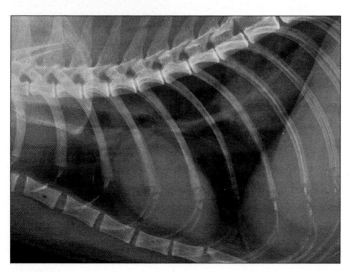

Figure 177

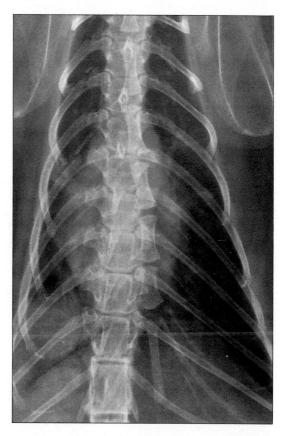

Figure 178

162 A 5-year-old neutered male domestic shorthair cat had progressive hindlimb ataxia over a period of 2–3 weeks. There was no apparent pain on palpation. Proprioception was reduced in both hindlimbs but muscle tone and reflexes were normal. Survey radiographs and a myelogram were obtained.

(a) Describe the lesion on the lateral survey radiograph (*Figure 179*) and lateral myelogram (*Figure 180*).
(b) What is your differential diagnosis?

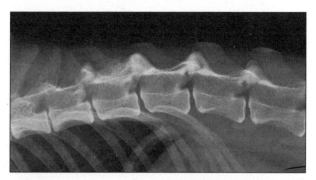

Figure 179

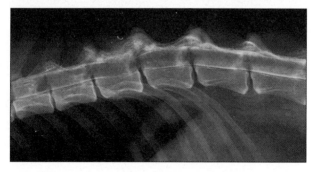

Figure 180

Head and Neck

163 What is the permanent dental formula of:

(a) The dog?
(b) The cat?

164 At what age is permanent dental eruption complete in the dog?

Figure 181

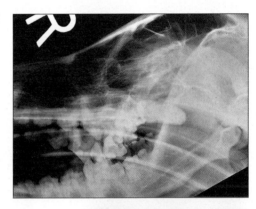

Figure 182

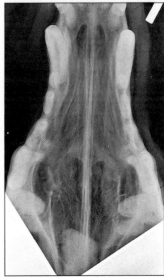

165 A 1-year-old female German shepherd dog had nasal discharge, noisy respiration and difficulty breathing for about 4 months. Physical examination did not indicate the diagnosis. Radiographs of the skull were obtained under general anaesthesia (*Figures 181* and *182*). What is your diagnosis?

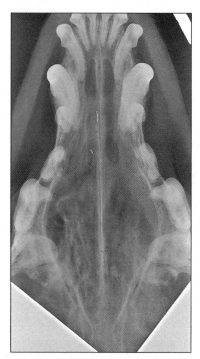

Figure 183

166 A 4-year-old male Jack Russell terrier had left-sided nasal discharge and occasional sneezing for 2 weeks. The discharge was mucoid with flecks of blood. Radiographs of the skull were obtained. What is your interpretation of the dorsoventral (intraoral) view of the nasal chambers shown in *Figure 183*?

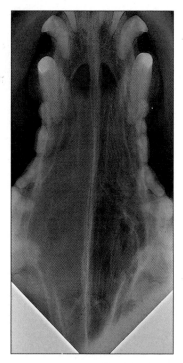

Figure 184

167 A 9-year-old retriever had nasal discharge and occasional sneezing for several weeks. Previous treatment using antibiotics produced some reduction in the amount of discharge, but this improvement was not maintained. Physical examination revealed a moderate mucopurulent, right-sided nasal discharge. Skull radiographs were obtained under anaesthesia. What is your interpretation of this dorsoventral (intraoral) view (*Figure 184*)?

168 An 11-year-old female domestic longhair cat had chronic left otitis externa. Response to medical management was limited, and total ear canal ablation was considered. Radiographs were obtained to evaluate the possibility of otitis media.

(a) Describe the abnormalities visible in *Figure 185*.
(b) What is your diagnosis?

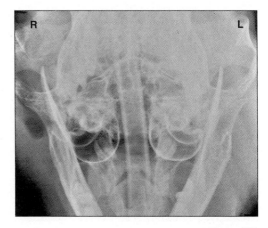

Figure 185

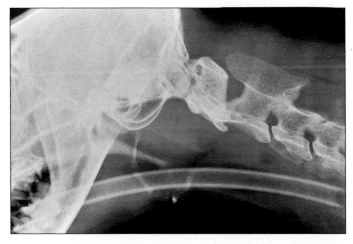

Figure 186

169 A 10-year-old female Siamese cat had weight loss, inappetance and polydipsia. Physical examination, including oral examination, revealed no abnormalities except for a swelling dorsal to the larynx. Before aspiration and biopsy of this swelling, a survey radiograph was obtained (*Figure 186*). Based on the location of the swelling, can you predict the aetiology?

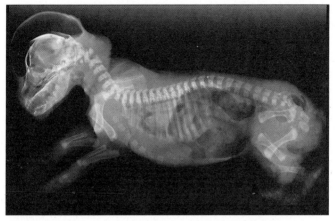

Figure 187

170 A 3-year-old cross-bred bitch had dystocia and needed a Caesarean operation to deliver the puppies, one of which was necrotic. Study the radiograph in *Figure 187* and list three signs of death.

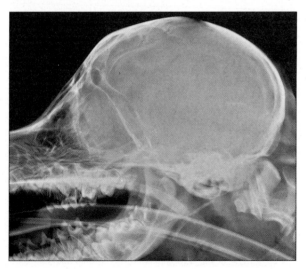

Figure 188

171 A 4-month-old male Dachshund had quadriparesis, proprioceptive deficits affecting all four limbs and abnormal behaviour including head shaking and compulsive pacing. Radiographs of the skull were obtained (*Figures 188* and *189*).

(a) Describe the abnormalities.
(b) What is your diagnosis?
(c) Name two additional diagnostic imaging methods that might confirm your diagnosis.

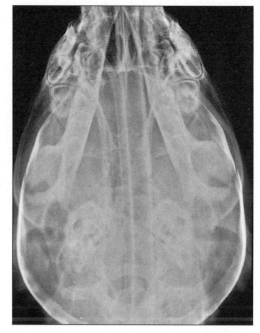

Figure 189

172 A 6-year-old male West Highland White terrier had blunt trauma to the left eye and intraocular haemorrhage. Blood in the anterior chamber prevented ophthalmoscopic examination. Ultrasonography was per-formed (*Figure 190*). What is your diagnosis?

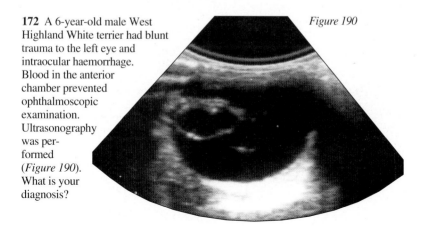

Figure 190

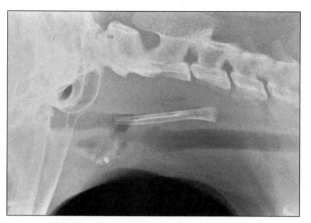

Figure 191

173 An old (formerly stray) neutered female cat had an acute onset of gagging, drooling and anorexia. The cat appeared distressed. Physical examination showed loss of several teeth and chronic periodontal disease but no other oral lesion to account for the clinical signs. The cat resented palpation of the pharyngeal/laryngeal area. The cat was sedated for endoscopy and a lateral cervical radiograph was obtained (*Figure 191*). What is your diagnosis? (Be precise.)

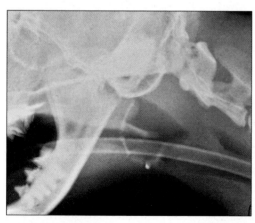

Figure 192

174 A 3-year-old neutered female domestic shorthair cat had bilateral mucoid nasal discharge and intermittent sneezing for about 2 weeks. The owner reported that the cat had no difficulty breathing, but it breathed by mouth during the examination. A lateral radiograph of the skull was obtained under anaesthesia (*Figure 192*).

(a) Describe the abnormality.
(b) What differential diagnoses would you consider?

175 *Figure 193* is a transverse image of a dog's head. What type of image is this?

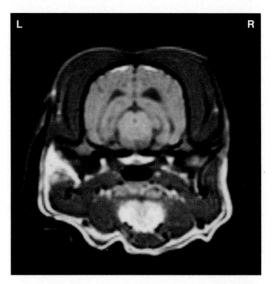

Figure 193

176 A 15-year-old Siamese cat gradually became withdrawn and aggressive and developed a tendency to circle to the left. X-ray computed tomography (CT) of the head was performed after administration of intravenous contrast medium.

(a) Describe the abnormalities on this transverse image (*Figure 194*).
(b) What is your diagnosis?

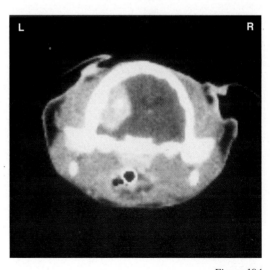

Figure 194

177 A 13-year-old female Siamese cat had polyphagia and weight loss. Physical examination revealed a single palpable thyroid nodule and a cardiac murmur. Serum thyroxine was elevated, confirming hyperthyroidism. ^{99m}Tc-pertechnetate thyroid scintigraphy was performed.

(a) Describe the abnormalities on the ventral view of the head and neck in *Figure 195*.
(b) What implications does the scan have for surgical treatment?

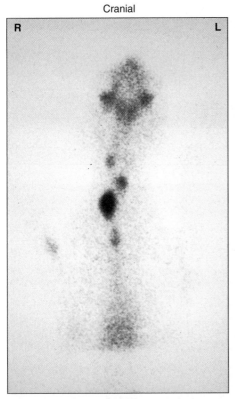

Cranial

R   L   *Figure 195*

Caudal

ANSWERS

Thorax

1 Photographic density (D) is defined as the logarithm of the ratio of light incident on the film (I_o) to light transmitted through the film (I_t), i.e.

$$D = \log I_o/I_t$$

Note that a dense area of the film is *dark*; this is one reason to avoid using the term 'density' for a lesion that appears light grey on a radiograph.

2 Opacity is the capacity of matter to obstruct the passage of radiation. When speaking about a radiograph it is a function of the attenuation of X-rays by an object. Opaque objects appear as white or light grey areas on a radiograph, and may be termed 'opacities' in a radiology report (Thrall, 1986).

3 ● Calcified tissue.
  ● Soft tissue/fluid.
  ● Fat.
  ● Gas.

4 The interface formed between:
(a) Soft tissue of the pericardium and air in the surrounding lung. Hence, if air in the lung is replaced by soft tissue or fluid, e.g. in bronchopneumonia, the heart may become invisible on radiographs.
(b) Soft tissue of the kidney and fat in the retroperitoneum. Hence, if an animal loses weight and its body fat deposits are reduced, the kidney may become invisible.

5 ● Voluntary patient movement, e.g. trying to sit up.
  ● Involuntary movement, e.g. breath motion.
  ● Cassette movement.
  ● X-ray tube head movement.
  ● Poor film–screen contact.

6 ● On many machines increasing the kVp will allow a reduced exposure time to be selected.
  ● This is a thin breed – it may be possible to remove the grid without significant loss of image quality, and this will allow a reduced exposure time.
  ● Reduce the film–focus distance.
  ● Interrupt the panting by attracting the dog's attention at the moment the exposure is made.
  ● Consider tranquilising or anaesthetising the dog.

7 (a) Double the mAs, by increasing either the mA or the exposure time.
  (b) Increase kVp by 10, a rule of thumb that works best in the range 70–80 kVp.

8 The mAs should be doubled. (The Bucky factor is the factor by which the exposure should be increased when using the grid).

9 (a) There is a large cranial mediastinal mass displacing the trachea dorsally and to the right. The heart is displaced caudally. Minor separation of the lung edges from the thoracic wall and loss of a clear ventral diaphragmatic outline indicate a small volume of pleural fluid.

(b) ● Lymphoma (common).
   ● Thymoma (rare).
   ● Haematoma.
Cytology of an aspirate of the mass indicated lymphoma.

10 (a) There is a large soft tissue mass in the left caudal thorax displacing the heart to the right. The ribs are unaffected, indicating that the mass is intrathoracic, probably pulmonary, in origin. Displacement of the heart (i.e. mediastinal shift) away from the lesion indicates that it is expansile.
(b) ● Primary lung tumour.
   ● Metastasis (usually multiple).
   ● Granuloma, which may be mycotic, heartworm-associated, or caused by a foreign body.
   ● Haematoma (rarely causes a well-defined mass).
   ● Abscess (rare).
   ● Cyst (rare).
The most common cause of a solitary lung mass is primary lung tumour. In this instance, the diagnosis was confirmed following fluoroscopically guided lung biopsy. The histological diagnosis was carcinoma.

Recognition of a mediastinal shift is important for diagnosis of lung opacities as it indicates whether a lesion is expansile, e.g. tumour (mediastinal shift *away* from the lesion), associated with reduced lung volume, i.e. collapsed lung lobe (mediastinal shift *towards* the lesion), or unassociated with changed lung volume, e.g. bronchopneumonia (usually causes no mediastinal shift). *Figure 196* shows the effect of an expansile mass (m), bronchopneumonia (centre) and lung lobe collapse (right)

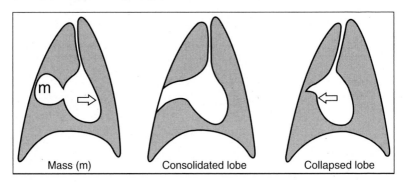

Mass (m)   Consolidated lobe   Collapsed lobe

Figure 196

11 On the *left* lateral. This is because identification of the mass depends largely on the presence of a clear soft tissue/air interface between it and the surrounding lung. This interface is less clear when air is expelled from the lung due to partial lung collapse on the dependent side of the animal, but the interface is preserved when the lesion is in the *non*-dependent lung (Biller and Myer, 1987).

12 On a lateral radiograph the ratio of the craniocaudal width of the heart to the distance between the cranial border of the fifth rib and caudal border of the seventh rib is normally 1.05 ± 0.07. In other words, the heart measures approximately two intercostal spaces wide. On a ventrodorsal radiograph the ratio of the maximum width of the heart to the width of the lung at the same level is normally 0.65 ± 0.06 (van den Broek and Darke, 1987).

13 (a) There is a moderately enlarged cardiac silhouette, enlarged pulmonary vessels and diffuse increase in lung opacity. The increased lung opacity is due to a diffuse interstitial infiltrate which is most marked dorsal to the heart base.
(b) The combination of abnormal heart size and lung infiltrate supports a diagnosis of left-sided cardiac failure. Ultrasonography indicated hypertrophic cardiomyopathy.

Left-sided cardiac failure producing pulmonary oedema in cats is now most often due to hypertrophic cardiomyopathy. Dilative cardiomyopathy is uncommon in cats fed on commercial cat foods (which include supplemental taurine), but is still seen in some cats fed on home-made food. Serum thyroxine levels should be determined in cats with cardiomyopathy to rule out hyperthyroidism as an underlying cause (Luis Fuentes, 1992).

14 (a) There is accumulation of opaque particulate material in a partially gas-filled viscus cranial to the heart (arrows) and there is ventral displacement of the trachea (T) (*Figure 197*). This represents a grossly dilated oesophagus draped over the trachea. As seen in other parts of the gastrointestinal tract, accumulation of opaque material ('gravel sign') occurs immediately cranial to a partial obstruction.

Why should there be a partial obstruction of the oesophagus at the level of the heart base in a young puppy?

Figure 197
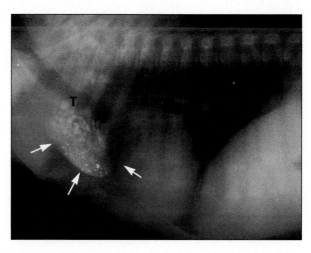

(b) Vascular ring anomaly. In this instance, the diagnosis was confirmed surgically and a persistent right aortic arch was repaired by ligating and dividing the ligamentum arteriosum, releasing the oesophagus. The prognosis is guarded in such animals because many do not regain adequate oesophageal function after surgery (Ellison, 1980).

15 ● Dysphagia or regurgitation not explained by survey radiographic findings.
   ● Investigation of a cervical swelling.
   ● Evaluation of the relationship of the oesophagus to a mediastinal lesion.
   ● Investigation of a cough associated with eating or other unexplained respiratory signs.

16 Suspected ruptured oesophagus. This is because water-soluble organic iodide contrast medium is less damaging to the cervical or mediastinal tissues than barium sulphate if extravasation occurs (Vessal *et al.,* 1975).

17 (a) Right-sided cardiac enlargement (*Figures 198* and *199*, small arrows), enlarged pulmonary artery segment visible on the dorsoventral view (*Figure 198*, large arrow) and attenuated pulmonary vasculature producing a hyperlucent lung. The radiographic signs indicate a right-sided cardiac lesion associated with pulmonary underperfusion.
(b) The radiographic signs are compatible with pulmonic stenosis (Fingland *et al.,* 1986) or tetralogy of Fallot. Pulmonic stenosis was confirmed using ultrasonography .

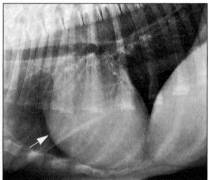

Figure 199

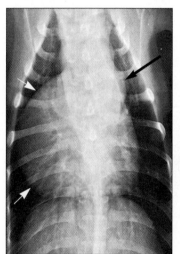

Figure 198

18 (a) Soft tissue masses are visible adjacent to the sternum (*Figure 200*, dotted arrow), overlying the cranial mediastinum (small arrows) and at the heart base (large arrow), compatible with enlargement of the sternal, mediastinal and tracheobronchial lymph nodes, respectively.
(b) Radiographic diagnosis: multiple enlarged lymph nodes; probable lymphoma.

   Lymphoma was confirmed by biopsy of a superficial lymph node. Recognition of lymph node enlargement on radiographs relies on knowledge of lymph node location. The radiograph in this animal shows the thoracic nodes that may be identified radiographically.

110

Figure 200

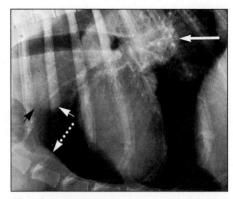

19 There is thickening of the bronchial walls, visible radiographically as parallel lines and thick rings throughout the lung. In general, bronchial thickening indicates chronic bronchitis but the underlying aetiology must be determined by means other than radiography, for example cytology and culture of bronchial washings (Padrid *et al.*, 1990).

The owner of this dog was a heavy smoker and seldom took the dog out for exercise. Hence, passive smoking is a potential cause of disease in this instance.

20 (a) Pleural fluid obscures the cardiac silhouette and separates the lung edges from the thoracic wall (*Figures 201* and *202,* arrows). The trachea and heart base are dorsally displaced. The fluid is relatively evenly distributed, with some accumulation around the left cranial lobe (dotted arrow). No lung lesion is visible.

Figure 201

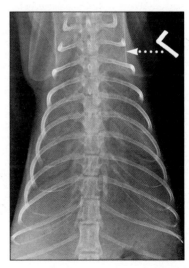

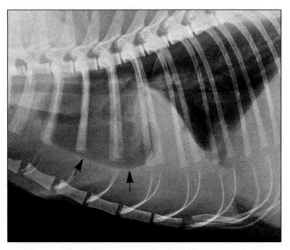

Figure 202

(b) The differential diagnosis of pleural fluid in a cat should include:
- Transudate secondary to heart failure, mediastinal mass, hypoproteinaemia or uraemia.
- Exudate secondary to pyothorax or viral disease (e.g. feline infectious peritonitis).
- Haemorrhage due to trauma.
- Chylothorax.

In this case, similar protein-containing (29 g/l) fluid with small numbers of neutrophils, lymphocytes and mesothelial cells was present in the pleural and peritoneal cavities. On serological tests the cat was positive for feline leukaemia virus and feline immunodeficiency virus. At postmortem examination lymphoid hyperplasia, pleuritis and peritonitis were found.

Despite the dorsally displaced trachea and heart base, no mediastinal mass or cardiomegaly was found at postmortem examination. The presence of fluid alone can cause displacement of these structures. This, and accumulation of pleural fluid around the cranial lung lobes, can mimic the radiographic appearance of a mediastinal mass or cardiomegaly (Snyder *et al.*, 1990). Repeating the radiographs after draining the pleural fluid, and/or ultrasonography may be necessary to establish the diagnosis (Konde and Spaulding, 1991).

21 (a) Fat separates the heart from the sternum on the lateral view. Soft tissue/fluid opacity obliterates normal lung detail on the right side. The right ventral portion of the diaphragm is also obscured and there is cranial displacement of the gastric antrum and spleen.
(b) Radiographic diagnosis: right-sided diaphragmatic rupture.
(c) Other techniques for confirming the diagnosis include upper gastrointestinal contrast series, positive contrast peritoneography (Rendano, 1979) and ultrasonography (Stowater and Lamb, 1989). The ultrasonograph in *Figure 203* is a transverse image of the liver in this case, showing normal demarcation (small arrows) between the liver (L) and lung on the left, but loss of the diaphragm on the right and cranial displacement of part of the liver (dotted arrow). This finding supports the radiographic diagnosis.

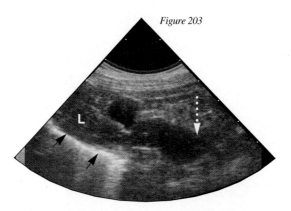

Figure 203

22 The lung edges are separated from the thoracic wall by a soft tissue/fluid opacity compatible with pleural fluid. Gas outlines the dorsal lung edge on the lateral view (white arrow), indicating small volume penumothorax; this may have occurred inadvertently at thoracocentesis.

There are two clues that this fluid is associated with a chronic pleuritis:
- Asymmetrical distribution, indicating that the fluid may be viscous or trapped by fibrinous/fibrous adhesions.
- Irregular lung margins on the lateral view (*Figure 204*, small arrows) compatible with pleural fibrosis/adhesions.

On the dorsoventral view (*Figure 205*) the left cranial lobe is small and irregular in outline but still contains air (dotted arrow). Reduced lung lobe volume usually is accompanied by increased opacity of the affected lobe and indicates collapse, i.e. loss of air. In this case, the continued presence of air in the lobe and its irregular outline indicate that reduced lung lobe size is due to contraction of the visceral pleura secondary to fibrosis. The lobe remains relatively well aerated and therefore is clearly visible through the pleural fluid.

Figure 204

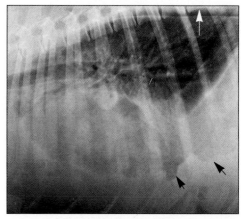

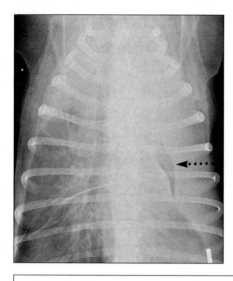

Figure 205

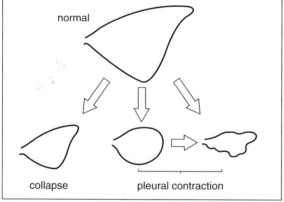

Figure 206

normal

collapse   pleural contraction

Figure 206 shows how the size and shape of a lung lobe may change in the presence of pleural fluid. As fluid (or gas) is introduced into the pleural space the lung lobe contracts. The lung lobe will tend to maintain its usual shape unless there is a specific reason for deformation, e.g. space-occupying mass or pleural fibrosis. The latter occurs in chronic pleuritis due to pyothorax or chylothorax and may produce rounded or irregular lung lobe borders (Fossum *et al.*, 1992; Schmidt and Wolvecamp, 1991).

In this case *Nocardia* sp. was cultured from the pleural fluid. Final diagnosis: *Nocardia* pyothorax.

23 (a) There is calcification of the lung, myocardium, aorta, abdominal arteries and gastric mucosa.

(b) These lesions represent 'metastatic calcification'. This occurs principally in kidney failure, but also in other causes of hypercalcaemia (Lamb *et al.*, 1991b). Metastatic calcium deposits usually cause no specific clinical signs; however, in this instance it seems plausible that the physical presence of the calcium deposits in the myocardium might ultimately reduce contractility or cause conduction disturbances.

24 (a) The cardiac silhouette is markedly enlarged, producing broad areas of sternal and diaphragmatic contact, and has an uneven opacity. The stomach is located more cranially than normal, indicating a small liver or cranial displacement of the liver. The seventh sternebra is foreshortened and the eighth is absent.

(b) This combination of radiographic signs is typical of congenital peritoneopericardial diaphragmatic hernia (Evans and Biery, 1980). In this instance the diagnosis was confirmed by ultrasonography, which showed part of the liver and spleen within the pericardial sac. In the absence of clinical signs referable to this lesion, the owners elected not to pursue surgical repair.

25 (a) The lung lesion is characterised by a patchy, asymmetrical lung infiltrate, which is most marked in the dorsal part of the right lung. The infiltrate is a mixed interstitial/alveolar type; air bronchograms are visible on the dorsoventral view.

(b) Differential diagnosis should include:
- Pulmonary haemorrhage and/or contusion.
- Pulmonary thromboembolism.
- Inhalation of foreign material.

The two commonest causes of alveolar infiltrates are bronchopneumonia, which usually affects the ventral lung, and pulmonary oedema, which usually produces a symmetrical infiltrate affecting the perihilar or caudodorsal lung. The lesion in this case is mainly dorsal and asymmetrical and, therefore, is atypical of either bronchopneumonia or oedema.

Asymmetrical lung infiltrate is often seen following haemorrhage, particularly that associated with trauma. Thromboembolism is another possibility; although uncommonly diagnosed radiographically, it should be considered, especially if known predisposing causes such as renal disease and hyperadrenocorticism are present. Finally, inhalation of smoke or foreign material may produce an asymmetrical lung infiltrate.

The dog died soon after the radiographs were obtained. Blood clotting tests were not performed. Postmortem examination revealed extensive pulmonary haemorrhage. Histopathology confirmed acute pulmonary haemorrhage but did not indicate the aetiology.

26 (a) There is cardiomegaly causing dorsal displacement of the trachea. Symmetrical, diffuse alveolar lung infiltrate is present, with air bronchograms in the caudal lobes. The cranial lobes have a less uniform alveolar infiltrate, compatible with air alveologram. Motion blur on the lateral view reflects rapid breathing.

(b) Differential diagnosis:
- Severe cardiogenic pulmonary oedema.
- Severe bronchopneumonia.
- Near-drowning.
- Smoke inhalation.

In this case the combined clinical and radiographic findings support severe cardiogenic pulmonary oedema. Ultrasonography revealed a dilated, hypocontractile left ventricle, compatible with dilative cardiomyopathy (Calvert *et al.*, 1982; Calvert and Brown, 1986). The dog died despite treatment.

Note that near-drowning and smoke inhalation are invariably suggested by the clinical history; these possiblities are included here only to provide a more complete differential diagnosis of the diffuse alveolar pattern.

27 (a) There is a patchy, heavy interstitial infiltrate mainly in the perihilar and ventral parts of the lung. The heart is obscured and cannot be adequately evaluated.
(b) Differential diagnosis should include:
- Bronchopneumonia.
- Inhalation pneumonia.
- Pulmonary haemorrhage.
- Cardiogenic pulmonary oedema.

The lung infiltrate in this case is predominantly ventral in distribution. In the dog this would strongly support some form of bronchopneumonia, but in the cat cardiogenic pulmonary oedema is variable in distribution and (as in this instance) can also occur in the ventral lung.

In this case, ultrasonography revealed hypertrophic cardiomyopathy. The heart often does not appear enlarged on radiographs because the concentric myocardial hypertrophy seen in this condition encroaches on the ventricle rather than increasing the external cardiac dimension, i.e.the cardiac silhouette. Serum thyroxine level was increased, indicating hyperthyroidism. The lung infiltrate cleared after treatment with frusemide.

When uncertainty exists about the cause of a lung infiltrate, the radiographs may be repeated after 12–24 hours of diuresis; a marked reduction in the lung infiltrate is usually apparent when oedema is the cause. Cellular infiltrates, e.g. in bronchopenumonia, are usually unaffected by diuresis. This is a useful test for pulmonary oedema, particularly if other facilities such as ultrasonography are unavailable.

28 (a) The lateral view (*Figure 207*) shows an opaque area of lung with faint air bronchograms (arrow) overlying the cardiac silhouette. A mediastinal blood vessel is visible (dotted arrow), indicating pneumomediastinum. The trachea is wide, reflecting increased inspiratory effort. The heart is narrow with a pointed apex, compatible with reduced blood volume, e.g. hypovolaemia due to shock.

Figure 207

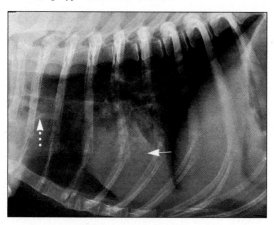

Figure 208

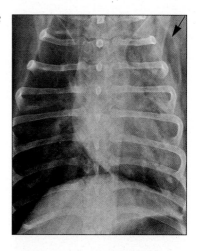

The ventrodorsal view (*Figure 208*) shows patchy increased opacity affecting the left lung and a mediastinal shift to the left. This combination of increased lung opacity and mediastinal shift towards the affected lung indicates reduced lung volume, i.e. collapse. Subcutaneous gas is visible near the left scapula (arrow).

(b) Radiographic diagnosis: left lung collapse; pneumomediastinum and subcutaneous gas; hypovolaemia.

Lateral displacement of the heart, i.e. mediastinal shift, has occurred in this case because the heart is pulled by negative pressure generated by the reduced lung volume (Lord and Gomez, 1985).

29 (a) The mitral valve leaflets are thick and nodular.

(b) The left atrium is approximately twice as large as the aortic root (the sizes are normally similar). Knowing the left ventricular dimensions enables calculation of fractional shortening (FS), using:

$$FS = LVD - LVS/LVD \times 100\%$$

In this instance FS = 41% (normal range 28–45%). FS should increase when afterload is reduced, e.g. in mitral insufficiency. Therefore, lack of an increase in the presence of mitral valve lesions and enlarged left atrium is evidence for poor myocardial function (Bonagura *et al.*, 1985).

Echocardiographic diagnosis: mitral insufficiency associated with nodular valvular lesions, probably endocardiosis; hypocontractile left ventricle, potential myocardial failure.

30 The heart is enlarged; the atria are prominent on the ventrodorsal view (*Figure 209, arrows*). The caudal vena cava is wide and kinked, and the pulmonary veins are enlarged and tortuous (*Figure 210*, small arrows), i.e. there is pulmonary congestion. There is no infiltrate to indicate pulmonary oedema.

Radiographic diagnosis: cardiomyopathy causing pulmonary and systemic congestion but not sufficiently decompensated to cause pulmonary oedema.

117

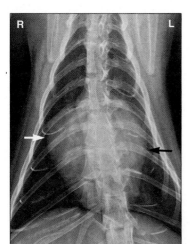

Figure 209

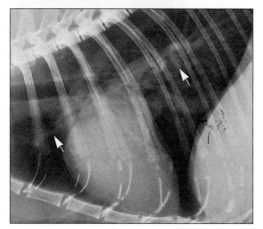

Figure 210

Ultrasonography confirmed hypertrophic cardiomyopathy with marked enlargement of the atria. Although enlargement of the atria indicates that end-diastolic pressure is increased, the absence of pulmonary oedema means that any increase blood volume has not yet exceeded the capacity of the pulmonary venous bed. Left atrial enlargement may be marked before pulmonary oedema develops when the progression of the underlying cardiac disease is slow.

31 ● Thymus (visible in puppies).
   ● Thymoma.
   ● Enlarged lymph node (e.g. lymphoma, lymphatic metastasis, granulomatous disease such as systemic mycosis).

- Other neoplasm (e.g. chemodectoma).
- Dilated oesophagus.
- Fat deposit.
- Haematoma.
- Ectopic thyroid gland mass (rare).

32 End-on pulmonary vessels:
- Never appear larger than the nearest longitudinal vessel.
- Are more opaque than longitudinal vessels of the same diameter.
- Become progressively smaller towards the periphery of the lung.

33 (a) There is a mild diffuse increase in lung opacity, which has the effect of smudging or obscuring the pulmonary vessels and caudal vena cava. This is an example of an interstitial pattern.
(b) ● Artefact, e.g. under-exposure, expiratory.
- 'Old dog lung'.
- Lymphoma.
- Diffuse pulmonary metastasis.
- Pneumonitis: viral (e.g. distemper); parasitic (e.g. *Dirofilaria, Angiostrongylus*); metabolic (e.g. uraemia, pancreatitis): inhalant (e.g. smoke, allergy); toxic (e.g. paraquat ingestion); idiopathic (e.g. pulmonary infiltrates with eosinophilia).
- Disease in transition: oedema; bronchopneumonia.

In this instance the dog had an acute onset of dyspnoea. Initial radiographs showed a diffuse alveolar pattern compatible with pulmonary oedema, which gradually resolved over the next 4 days. There were no signs of cardiac disease; the oedema was thought to represent an allergic or anaphylactic reaction, although no definite diagnosis was made. This radiograph was obtained 3 days after the start of clinical signs and shows residual, clearing oedema.

34 The oesophagus is dilated with gas *(Figure 211*, arrowheads) and overlying the heart is an area of alveolar infiltrate with air bronchograms (arrow).

Figure 211

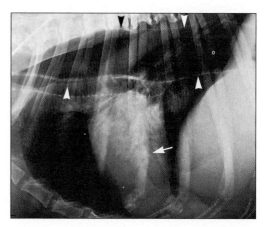

Radiographic diagnosis: megaoesophagus and aspiration pneumonia. Aspiration pneumonia is a common finding in combination with megaoesophagus. As in this case, the lesion is often localised to the caudoventral lung field and overlaps the heart on a lateral view. The right middle lobe is most often affected, hence the lung lesion is most visible on a *left* lateral view. A ventrodorsal view is also recommended for evaluation of the ventral lung field in potential bronchopneumonia cases.

Whenever megaoesophagus is identified, it is important to look for signs of aspiration pneumonia. Conversely, when ventral lung consolidation is identified, look for megaoesophagus.

35 (a) There is a diffuse alveolar infiltrate affecting the entire lung. Gaseous dilatation of the stomach reflects hyperpnoea.
(b) Diffuse lung oedema is sometimes found in animals with diseases affecting the central nervous system, such as epilepsy, electrocution or hypoglycaemia. The typical radiographic appearance is a bilaterally symmetrical alveolar infiltrate mainly affecting the caudal lobes (Lord, 1975). The exact pathogenesis is not established but it is thought that the brain lesion leads to overstimulation of sympatheticoadrenal activity, which in turn causes a sudden shift of blood from the systemic to the pulmonary circulation. At the same time, adrenergic discharges limit left ventricular diastolic filling, hence end-diastolic pressure rises acutely and pulmonary oedema follows.

In this instance, the final diagnosis was a dry (non-effusive) form of feline infectious peritonitis affecting the brain.

36 (a) The thoracic radiograph shows multiple, variously sized nodules scattered throughout the lung fields. The heart is small for this breed and the pulmonary vessels and caudal vena cava are reduced in calibre, indicating hypovolaemia. The abdominal radiograph shows diffuse loss of serosal detail and blotchy opacity. A relatively homogeneous area is seen cranioventrally, raising the possibility of a mass in the spleen.
(b) Radiographic diagnosis: pulmonary metastasis; possible splenic mass; peritoneal fluid and/or peritoneal adhesions/carcinomatosis.

A splenic neoplasm, multiple nodules in the peritoneum and omentum, and haemoperitoneum were found at laparotomy. The histological diagnosis was haemangiosarcoma.

This case illustrates the classic presentation of haemangiosarcoma of the spleen. The combination of this breed, age, anaemia and haemoperitoneum make this diagnosis very likely (Prymak *et al.*, 1988). The radiographic findings also support this diagnosis and indicate that metastasis has already occurred.

37 (a) Well-defined, bubbly or segmented-appearing opaque lines are visible in the area of the caudal segment of the left cranial lobe. These appear to originate at the hilum and branch peripherally. They represent grossly enlarged and distorted bronchial walls. Less prominent lesions also affect the bronchi on the right and dorsally.
(b) Radiographic diagnosis: bronchiectasis (Myer and Burk, 1973).

38 (a) There is a large-volume pneumothorax on the left, associated with caudal displacement of the left hemidiaphragm and mediastinal shift to the right. There is bilateral lung lobe collapse with aerated lung visible only in the right caudal lobe.
(b) This pneumothorax is apparently unilateral. Furthermore, the mediastinal shift towards the contralateral side indicates that there is increased pleural pressure on the left, i.e. this is a *tension* pneumothorax.

(c) Most cats or dogs with pneumothorax have air in both sides of the pleural cavity and, even if the distribution of air is asymmetrical, show no mediastinal shift. Unless there is a large volume of pleural air causing dyspnoea, treatment may be conservative, i.e. allowing the air to resorb naturally. However, tension penumothorax can progress rapidly to cardiorespiratory collapse and death. It must be recognised and treated promptly by aspirating the pleural air and monitoring for recurrence.

39 (a) The cardiac silhouette is partially obscured and there are prominent pleural fissure lines indicating pleural fluid. Overlying the caudoventral thorax on the right lateral view are smoothly marginated gas lucencies which appear tubular (*Figure 213*, arrows) ; on the left lateral view (*Figure 212*) a round gas lucency is visible.

Figure 212

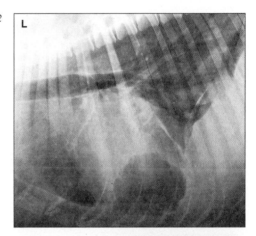

Figure 213

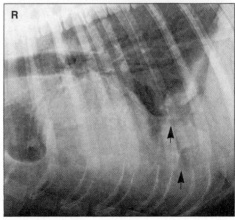

(b) The differential diagnosis should include pneumohaemothorax and diaphragmatic rupture.

Ultrasonography of the cranial abdomen showed that the liver and stomach were in normal positions caudal to an intact diaphragm. Thoracocentesis produced 10 ml of bloody fluid and froth. *Diagnosis:* pneumohaemothorax.

It is not uncommon for traumatised dogs to have radiographic signs of pleural fluid and gas. In such instances, pleural gas may form bubbles of various shapes, sometimes simulating a gas-filled viscus and inviting the misdiagnosis of diaphragmatic rupture. Ultrasonography is a useful means of examining the diaphragm in such cases; when it is not available, other radiographic projections (such as ventrodorsal) or peritoneography can provide evidence that the diaphragm is intact. Removing the pleural fluid and repeating the radiographs should also be considered. Do not hurry to take these cases to surgery.

In this instance repeat thoracic radiographs, including a ventrodorsal, were obtained after thoracocentesis and 24-hour observation and were within normal limits.

40 (a) There is marked cardiomegaly causing elevation of the trachea and increased craniocaudal dimension of the heart. The enlarged left atrium is visible (*Figure 214*, small arrows) although it is partially obscured by infiltrate in the caudal lung lobes. The caudal cervical trachea is narrow due to infolding of the dorsal membrane (large arrow). Hence, the principal abnormalities are:
- Tracheal collapse.
- Cardiomegaly.
- Pulmonary oedema.

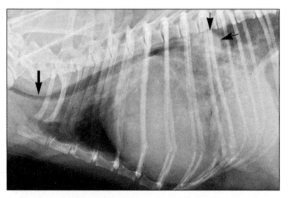

Figure 214

(b) These abnormalities are related in the sense that they are both very common in small breeds of dog and therefore often occur together. The synergistic effect of the tracheal, cardiac and pulmonary lesions compounds the respiratory difficulty. Any additional stress such as hot weather or excitement can precipitate an acute crisis (Dallman *et al.*, 1988).

The diagnosis of tracheal collapse may be made with confidence from a lateral view when it is recognised that the curved border overlying the dorsal aspect of the trachea is a gas/soft tissue interface, i.e. it represents an infolding of the dorsal tracheal membrane that narrows the tracheal lumen. *Figure 215* correlates the change in appearance of the trachea on a lateral radiograph with changes in its cross-sectional appearance. Note that as the oesophagus is not visible radiographically (unless there is pneumomediastinum or the oesophagus is filled with

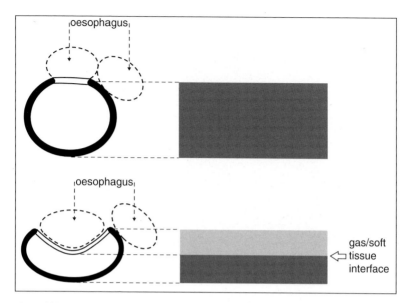

Figure 215

gas or contrast medium), changes in its position cannot mimic tracheal collapse. The oesophagus may be dorsal or lateral to the trachea. Admittedly, a full oesophagus lying dorsal to the trachea may *exacerbate* the collapse, but it does not represent the *cause* of the radiographic appearance.

Mild infolding of the dorsal tracheal membrane is sometimes visible on lateral thoracic radiographs of large breeds of dogs that do not suffer tracheal collapse. In these instances it represents a normal physiological effect of reduced tracheal air pressure during deep or forceful inspiration.

41 (a) This is an example of a pneumopericardiogram (*Figure 216*). A catheter (white arrow) has been inserted into the pericardial cavity, and any fluid present has been withdrawn and replaced by air.
(b) A rounded soft tissue mass (M) is outlined by the pericardial air on the craniodorsal aspect of the heart. The adjacent border of the heart is indented by the mass (black arrows).
(c) The principal differential diagnoses are right atrial haemangiosarcoma and heart-base neoplasm, e.g. chemodectoma, ectopic thyroid neoplasm.

Pneumopericardiography has been described as an aid to the diagnosis of pericardial fluid in dogs (Thomas *et al.,* 1984). Ultrasonography is a less invasive method for detection of pericardial fluid and also has the potential to identify the underlying cause. However, pneumopericardiography should be considered if ultrasonography is unavailable or if the results are not diagnostic. Insufflation for pneumopericardiography may be combined with therapeutic removal of fluid.

When a mass is identified in the area of the right atrium, it is important also to examine the abdomen because of the potential for multicentric or metastatic haemangiosarcoma to be present in both sites (Waters *et al.,* 1988).

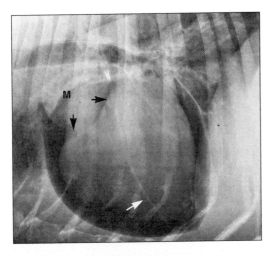

Figure 216

42 ● Interstitial or alveolar lung infiltrate.
  ● Enlarged hilar lymph nodes.
  ● Pleural fluid.
    (Ackerman and Spencer, 1982.)

43 Pulmonary histoplasmosis (Burk *et al.*, 1978).

44 ● Enlarged right ventricle.
  ● Enlarged main pulmonary artery.
  ● Enlarged, tortuous, or blunted peripheral pulmonary artery branches.
  ● Lung infiltrate – diffuse interstitial, nodular or alveolar.
  ● Signs of right heart failure (e.g. hepatomegaly, ascites).
    (Ackerman, 1987.)

45 Differential diagnosis of pericardial fluid in small animals (in approximate order of prevalence).

Dog	*Cat*
Neoplasia, e.g. haemangiosarcoma, chemodectoma, metastasis	Infection, e.g. feline infectious peritonitis
Idiopathic	Cardiomyopathy
Congestive heart failure	Lymphoma
Ruptured left atrium	Metastasis
Trauma	Uraemia
Coagulopathy	Coagulopathy
Infection, e.g. mycotic	
Uraemia	
Pericardial cyst	

(Berg and Wingfield, 1984; Rush *et al.*, 1990.)

46 (a) There is a large, clearly marginated soft tissue mass containing a small amount of gas in the caudodorsal mediastinum. This is associated with dilatation of the oesophagus and caudal displacement of the dorsal part of the diaphragm. The gastric silhouette is abnormally small.
(b) Radiographic diagnosis: hiatal hernia.

An important part of the interpretation in this case is recognition that the large mass is in the mediastinum. This is a fairly safe conclusion to reach when a large intrathoracic mass is centered exactly on the midline and is associated with an oesophageal abnormalitiy. In this instance it was considered unnecessary to confirm the diagnosis by oesophagography and the dog had surgery to correct the defect. The Shar-pei is a breed predisposed to hiatal hernia (Bright *et al.*, 1990).

47 (a) There is a poorly circumscribed, local interstitial infiltrate in the middle of the right caudal lobe (*Figures 217* and *218,* arrows). The location of the infiltrate indicates that it may be associated with the principal bronchus.
(b) ● Localised bronchitis, e.g. associated with inhaled foreign body.
   ● Localised haemorrhage.
   ● Infarct/embolism.

Figure 217

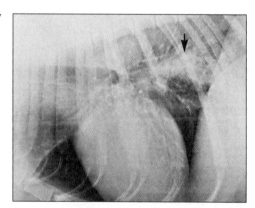

Figure 218

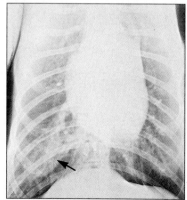

(c) Given the peribronchial location, bronchoscopy offers an attractive, relatively non-invasive means of further evaluating this area. Bronchoscopy using a flexible fibreoptic endoscope revealed an ear of corn and purulent exudate in the right caudal lobe bronchus.

Bronchial foreign bodies may be identified directly on thoracic radiographs when they appear opaque, but many are not opaque (e.g. plant seeds or fragments or twigs), and are recognisable indirectly by the peribronchial infiltrate they induce (Dobbie *et al.,* 1986). In cases where the bronchus is obstructed, complete lobar consolidation and collapse occur.

48 (a) A large mass on the dorsal midline displaces the trachea ventrally and to the right. The position of the mass indicates that it is mediastinal in origin.
(b) ● Oesophageal lesion, e.g. dilatation due to foreign body, mass.
   ● Aortic lesion, e.g. neoplasm, aneurysm.
   ● Other mediastinal neoplasm, e.g. lymphoma, haemangiosarcoma.
   ● Haematoma.
   ● Abscess.
   ● Cyst.
An oesophagram (not shown) revealed displacement of the oesophagus around the mass, ruling out a primary oesophageal lesion. The final diagnosis, based on biopsy, was chemodectoma, probably of aortic origin. Masses in the craniodorsal mediastinum are uncommon (Mitten, 1982).

49 ● Primary lung tumour.
   ● Metastasis.
   ● Mycotic granuloma, e.g. blastomycosis.
   ● *Paragonimus* sp. infection.
   ● Abscess.
   ● Partially fluid-filled lung bulla.
   ● Partially fluid-filled cyst.

50 ● *Diffuse:* overexposure; weight loss; hypovolaemia; overinflation; air trapping; emphysema.
   ● *Focal:* bulla (congenital or traumatic); lobar emphysema; thromboembolism.

Abdomen

51 There is considerable inter-breed variation in radiographic liver size, so it is not possible to give simple criteria for normal. However, in normal deep-chested dogs in left lateral recumbence the distance from the most cranial part of the dome of the diaphragm to the caudoventral tip of the liver, compared with the length of the eleventh thoracic vertebral body (T11), is 6.1 ($\pm$0.8) $\times$ T11. This distance appears to correlate well with liver volume in normal dogs and could be used as an aid to recognition of symmetrical increases or decreases in hepatic volume (van Bree and Sackx, 1987).

52 Generalised splenomegaly:
- Iatrogenic, e.g. due to barbiturates or phenothiazine administration.
- Infiltrative diseases, e.g. lymphoma, histoplasmosis.
- Lymphoid hyperplasia.
- Chronic anaemia.
- Vascular stasis, e.g. congestion due to splenic torsion or gastric torsion.

53 (a) In dogs the length of the kidneys on a ventrodorsal view, compared with the length of the second lumbar vertebral body (L2), is normally 3.04 ($\pm$0.22) $\times$ L2 (Feeney, 1977).
(b) In cats the kidneys are slightly asymmetrical; the right normally measures 2.95 ($\pm$0.04) $\times$ L2, the left 2.46 ($\pm$0.05) $\times$ L2 (Barrett and Kneller, 1972).

54 (a) The stomach and large intestine are full, preventing adequate examination of the intra-abdominal structures.
(b) A repeat survey radiograph was obtained after a 24-hour fast and an enema to empty the large intestine. This procedure was not completely successful but a spherical mass (M) is now clearly visible dorsal to the spleen (*Figure 219*, p.128). Ultrasound-guided biopsy of the mass was performed. Histology indicated splenic haemangiosarcoma.
   This case illustrates the value of proper patient preparation before radiography. The time taken to let the intestinal tract empty, to empty a full bladder, or to sedate a dog to improve positioning, is often rewarded with a correct diagnosis.

55 The spleen is enlarged.
   The spleen is not usually visible on a lateral abdominal radiograph of a cat. In this instance it produces a broad silhouette and, although there are no useful quantitative criteria for spleen size in the cat or dog to support this interpretation, the spleen is probably enlarged.
   Splenomegaly in the cat is commonly associated with lymphoma; this diagnosis was confirmed after bone marrow biopsy.

56 The ventrodorsal abdominal radiograph shows caudal displacement of the lesser curvature of the stomach (*Figure 220*, p.128, arrows) compatible with a mass in the liver or a gastric mural lesion. Poor abdominal detail in this instance is accentuated by a wet hair coat, which produces an overlying streaky artefact. Ultrasonography revealed a 3.6 cm-diameter hyperechoic mass in the liver adjacent to the stomach. The histological diagnosis was hepatocellular carcinoma.
   Displacement of the stomach is the commonest radiographic sign of liver neoplasia in the dog (Evans, 1987). Ultrasonography was useful in this instance not because it provided a specific diagnosis but because it confirmed and explained the radiographic lesion and provided guidance for biopsy.

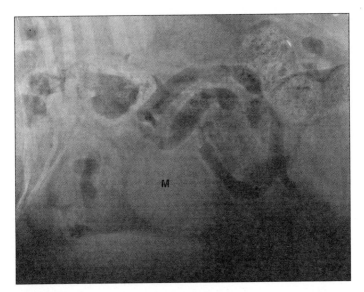

Figure 219

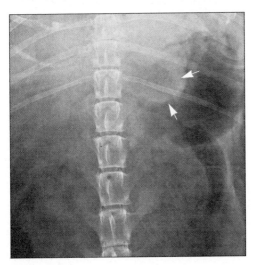

Figure 220

57 (a) There is multifocal calcification of the hepatic parenchyma.

(b) Calcification of the liver has been associated with a variety of chronic hepatic diseases. In many animals calcification represents the remains of an inactive lesion, such as an abscess, or is associated with hepatic nodular hyperplasia and is not clinically significant. However, in a few animals it does represent an active lesion (Lamb *et al.*, 1991b).

Liver biopsy in this instance showed severe, suppurative inflammation of the biliary tract with extension into the hepatic parenchyma, microabscessation and calcification. The final diagnosis was severe ascending cholangiohepatitis. This was considered to be the cause of the clinical and radiographic signs.

58 (a) The survey radiograph shows a predominantly fluid-filled, non-distended small intestine. The contrast study shows rapid intestinal transit, evidence of thickened intestinal wall, and dilution of barium suspension in the rectum.

(b) This combination of signs is typical of enteritis.

Do not misinterpret the rough appearance of the contrast margin in the small intestine. This appearance, sometimes called 'pavingstone' or 'cobblestone' is a normal variant (Morgan, 1981).

59 (a) The thoracic radiograph (*Figure 221*) shows enlargement of the sternal lymph node (arrow). On the abdominal radiograph (*Figure 222*) there is a gas-filled, thickened, corrugated-appearing portion of small intestine in the mid-ventral abdomen (arrows); there is reduced serosal detail in the area of the intestinal lesion.

(b) The abdominal radiograph is compatible with a focal small intestinal mural lesion, possibly with local peritonitis and/or fluid accumulation. Enlargement of the sternal lymph node (which drains the peritoneal cavity) is compatible with metastasis.

A jejunal neoplasm with adherent omentum and enlarged mesenteric lymph nodes were found at laparotomy and the dog was destroyed. A histological diagnosis was not obtained.

The finding of a localised, irregular or corrugated gas lucency associated with intestinal neoplasia has been described in a review of caecal neoplasms (Gibbons and Murtaugh,1990).

Figure 221

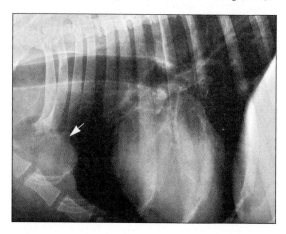

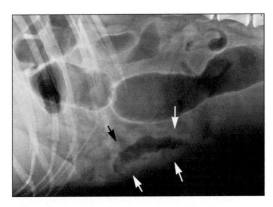
Figure 222

60 Ventral mid-abdominal mass in the male dog:
- Splenic neoplasm.
- Intestinal mass, e.g. neoplasm, foreign body.
- Pancreatic mass, e.g. pseudocyst.
- Mesenteric mass, e.g. lipoma, abscess.
- Abdominal wall mass, e.g. mesothelioma.
- Paraprostatic cyst.
- Retained testicle.

61 Both lateral views show localised dilatation of part of the small intestine. Two dilated loops are visible cranial to the urinary bladder; in one view their lumen contains gas, in the other, two round opacities are seen. The degree of dilatation (diameter of affected small intestine is greater than L2) supports obstruction (Gibbs and Pearson, 1973; McNeel, 1986), but do not be tempted to assume that the two round opacities are foreign bodies. They do not persist and simply represent fluid-filled intestine seen end on. Radiographic diagnosis: small intestinal obstruction.

Laparotomy confirmed total obstruction of the mid-jejunum caused by a piece of rubber. The jejunum was reddened, with small pieces of adherent fibrin, and there was a small amount of peritoneal fluid.

62 (a) There is a distended portion of the small intestine (diameter almost twice the length of L2) which contains accumulated opaque particulate material and gas. Abdominal serosal detail is normal. Incidental finding of spondylosis deformans.
(b) Radiographic diagnosis: partial obstruction of the small intestine, cause not identified.

This is an example of the 'gravel sign' of partial obstruction, whereby non-digestible material (often opaque, e.g. bone fragments) accumulates immediately proximal to a narrow, non-distensible intestinal lesion. Any circumferential mural thickening of the intestinal wall could produce a partial obstruction, but neoplasia is the most common aetiology (Gibbs and Pearson, 1986).

In this case, a mid-jejunal neoplasm was confirmed at laparotomy and was resected. Multiple nodules were found in the liver. The histological diagnosis was adenocarcinoma with metastasis to the liver.

63 (a) There is extreme gaseous dilatation of part of the intestine. The size of the distended portion supports large intestine, but the location is abnormal. The barium enema shows filling

only of the rectum. Attempts to fill more of the intestine were unsuccessful.
(b) Radiographic diagnosis: atresia coli.

The kitten was destroyed and the diagnosis confirmed at postmortem examination. There was no connection between the distended, blind-ended large intestine and vestigial rectum. Peritoneal fluid contributed to the abdominal distension.

64 (a) The radiographs show a sausage-shaped soft tissue mass within the descending large intestine (*Figures 223* and *224,* arrows). The small intestine contains fluid and some bubbles but is not distended. The ultrasound scan shows the cross-sectional view of a portion of intestine and fat *within* the large intestine. The radiographic and ultrasonographic findings indicate intussusception (Penninck *et al.*, 1990).

Figure 223

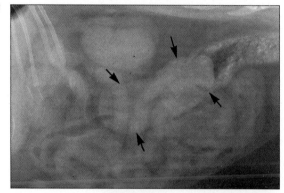

Figure 224

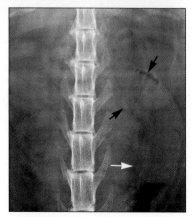

(b) The prognosis is guarded when an older dog or cat has intussusception, because of the potential for an intestinal neoplasm to act as an initiating factor. In this case, the intussusception could not be reduced fully and was resected. Histological examination indicated peritoneal fibrosis and mild granulomatous inflammation but no evidence of a specific initiating cause.

65 Bilaterally enlarged kidneys in the dog:
- Polycystic kidney disease.
- Hydronephrosis.
- Infiltrative diseases, e.g. lymphoma.
- Acute nephritis, e.g. leptospirosis.
- Compensatory hypertrophy, e.g. in congenital portosystemic shunts.
- Subcapsular fluid accumulation, e.g. haemorrhage.

66 Asymmetrical kidney size in the cat:
(a) The large kidney:
- Compensatory hypertrophy.
- Unilateral kidney disease, e.g. hydronephrosis, neoplasia (e.g. lymphoma), abscess, cyst, subcapsular fluid (e.g. haemorrhage, extravasated urine, inflammatory exudate, e.g. in feline infectious peritonitis).
(b) The small kidney:
- Hypoplasia.
- Chronic renal disease with fibrosis, e.g. pyelonephritis, glomerulonephritis.

67 On a lateral abdominal radiograph the ventrodorsal dimension of the prostate may be compared to the distance from the ventral aspect of the sacral promontory to the cranial aspect of the pubic bone, i.e. the pelvic inlet. The normal ratio between these measurements is 0.56 ($\pm$0.04). In other words, a normal prostate measures no more than 60% of the pelvic inlet (Feeney *et al.*, 1987).

68 Calcified prostate lesions:
- Neoplasia, e.g. adenocarcinoma.
- Chronic prostatitis.
- Prostatic cyst (intraprostatic or paraprostatic).
- Urethral calculus superimposed on the prostate.

69 Normal dogs often show a small amount of prostatic reflux during urethrography. Large amounts of reflux are more likely to be associated with disease but there is no apparent correlation between the amount of reflux and the type of disease (Thrall, 1981).

70 Radiolucent filling defects on cystography:
- Urolith.
- Soft tissue mass, e.g. neoplasm, polypoid cystitis lesion.
- Ureterocoele.
- Blood clot.
- Air bubble.
- Foreign body (rare).

71 Indications for intravenous urography:
- To identify the kidneys and ureters if they are not visible on survey radiographs.
- Normal survey radiographs in an animal with clinical signs of kidney disease.
- Abnormal kidney size or shape.
- Mass in the area of the kidney or ureter.
- Suspected ectopic ureter.
- To investigate the origin of urinary tract haemorrhage.
- To provide a crude estimate of relative kidney function in suspected unilateral kidney disease.

72 (a) The mid-pelvic urethra is wide and contains an oval filling defect, apparently attached to the dorsal urethral mucosa. The vagina appears normal.

(b) Radiographic diagnosis: urethral neoplasm.

Transitional cell carcinoma is the most common neoplasm in this location. It often produces radiographic signs of extensive invasion of the urethral mucosa.lesion (Davies and Read, 1990; Moroff *et al.*, 1991). In this case, the localised mucosal attachment, intraluminal location and rounded shape support a polypoid, possibly benign, lesion such as leiomyoma.

In this instance permission was not given to attempt surgical treatment and no definitive diagnosis was made. However, this case does illustrate the use of vaginourethrography and the fact that blood pooling in the vagina can occur secondary to a urethral lesion.

73 (a) There is prostatomegaly (P) and a localised fringe of periosteal new bone on the ventral aspect of the body of L6 *(Figure 225*, arrow).

(b) Radiographic diagnosis: probable prostatic carcinoma with metastasis to the lumbar spine.

This combination of clinical and radiographic signs is characteristic of prostatic carcinoma. There are few other conditions that can produce the bone lesion (for example, primary bone tumour or bacterial osteomyelitis) and these are unlikely to also cause clinical signs of prostate disease.

Ultrasonography in this instance revealed a 4.9 cm-diameter gland, with heterogeneous echotexture comprising hypoechoic and hyperechoic areas and possibly a cavitary lesion. The ultrasonographic findings confirmed the presence of prostate disease; however, because ultrasonographic findings in prostatic carcinoma are non-specific (Feeney *et al.*, 1987) it is advisable to base the diagnosis on the results of biopsy.

Figure 225

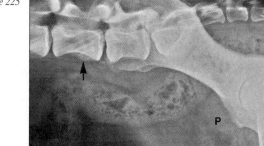

74 (a) Contrast medium has extravasated in the right retroperitoneum, the right pelvis and proximal ureter are dilated, and the urinary bladder mis-shapen. Reduced serosal detail is still apparent, although contrast medium is not visible in the peritoneal cavity.

(b) The radiographic diagnosis is a ruptured right ureter. The mis-shapen urinary bladder could indicate partial or complete rupture that has sealed spontaneously. The peritoneal fluid could be urine from a bladder rupture or haemorrhage.

A laparotomy was performed and the right kidney and ruptured ureter were removed. Blood-stained urine was present in the peritoneal cavity. The bladder was bruised and had an adherent fibrinous clot on its cranial aspect but it was not leaking.

Urinary tract damage commonly occurs in dogs and cats in cases of abdominal or pelvic trauma. In a radiographic study of 100 dogs with pelvic fractures (Selcer, 1982) 39 had urinary tract damage including avulsion of a ureter, ruptured bladder, haemorrhage into the bladder, ruptured urethra, herniation of the bladder and hydroureter/hydronephrosis. There were no clinical signs suggesting urinary tract damage in 13 of 39 (33%) of these cases, emphasising the importance of careful radiographic examination to identify these injuries.

75 (a) The right kidney is small and irregular in shape. It contains radiating zones of calcification in the medulla, probably involving the tubules or collecting ducts. These lesions are most visible on the postmortem radiograph shown in *Figure 226*. The left kidney appears normal in size, shape and opacity.
(b) Radiographic diagnosis: end-stage disease of the right kidney. Although the left kidney appears normal, the elevated serum creatinine indicates that it must also be diseased.

Histology confirmed renal scarring, glomerulosclerosis, tubular atrophy and chronic inflammatory cell infiltrate but the underlying aetiology could not be determined.

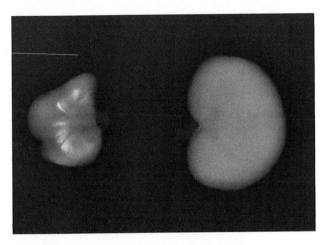

Figure 226

76 (a) There is a large soft tissue mass with calcification radiating out from its centre occupying the right dorsal abdomen. This is the normal position for the right kidney but the right kidney is not visible. The mass is therefore likely to be an abnormal right kidney. The intestine is displaced caudally and to the left by the mass, and the lateral view shows that the stomach is compressed. Serosal detail is good; the left kidney appears normal.
(b) Differential diagnosis:
 ● Kidney tumour.
 ● Osseous metaplasia of the renal pelvis.
Other possible causes of severe unilateral kidney enlargement (such as cyst or abscess) were considered unlikely because the appearance of the calcification spreading out from the centre of the lesion indicates a solid expansile mass rather than a cavitary lesion.

Core biopsies of the mass were obtained under ultrasound guidance. Histology indicated sarcoma, probably myxosarcoma. A needle was directed into the centre of the mass and a straw-coloured acellular fluid compatible with urine was obtained . The owners elected not to pursue treatment and the dog was destroyed without permission for postmortem examination.

Kidney neoplasia is relatively uncommon in dogs (Moulton, 1990); osseous metaplasia of the renal pelvis is *rare* (Miller and Sande, 1980).

77 There is moderate dilatation of a large proportion of the small intestine; the diameter of certain loops is similar to the length of L2 (*Figure 227*, arrows). The intestinal content is mainly fluid. In the caudodorsal abdomen a roughly circular, well-defined gas lucency is visible (arrowheads) around a soft tissue structure which contains a fine lucent line. This appearance is characteristic of a foreign body (in this case a fruit seed). The fine line dividing the seed indicates that it is a dicotyledon!

Radiographic diagnosis: distal small intestinal obstruction due to foreign body (fruit seed). A chestnut was removed at laparotomy.

A number of common fruit seeds may cause intestinal obstruction. These are usually visible on good-quality radiographs and may be recognised by their round or oval shape and by gas around or within the shell (Mayrhofer, 1985). With practice these may be readily identified on radiographs.

Identification of a foreign body is a helpful indication for exploratory surgery, particularly when other radiographic signs of obstruction are not convincing. For example, when the obstructing material is lodged in the duodenum or proximal jejunum, the intestine may not dilate because vomiting removes any excess fluid.

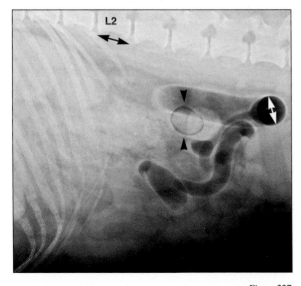

Figure 227

78 (a) On each radiograph (*Figures 228* and *229*) there is a localised mottled gas lucency overlying the liver (arrows). The location, close to the diaphragm and to the right of midline, is compatible with the gallbladder. The clear visualisation of the serosal surface of the stomach (dotted arrow) indicates pneumoperitoneum.

(b) Radiographic diagnosis: hepatic abscess or emphysematous cholecystitis; pneumoperitoneum may reflect rupture of a visceral structure such as the hepatic duct or intestine.

The dog died 2 days later. Postmortem examination confirmed hepatic abscess secondary to severe cholecystitis, ruptured gallbladder and peritonitis.

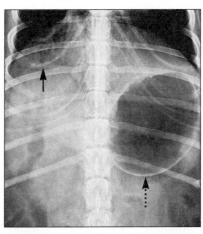

Figure 228

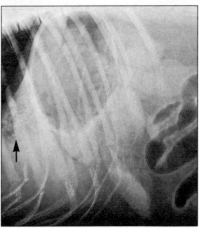

Figure 229

Gas in the liver is an uncommon radiographic finding (Lord *et al.*, 1982). It can occur in three ways:

- Gas in the gallbladder associated with severe cholecystitis (can occur in diabetes mellitus).
- Gas in hepatic parenchyma caused by necrosis or abscessation.
- Gas in the portal veins secondary to gastric or intestinal ischaemia (sometimes seen following gastric torsion).

79 (a) There is mild spondylosis deformans in the lumbar spine and a poorly circumscribed area of increased opacity, and loss of serosal detail in the mid-dorsal abdomen. There is no convincing 'mass effect.'
(b) This appearance might be produced by a disease that causes local fluid accumulation in the mesentery or peritoneal cavity and/or thickening of the mesentery and peritoneum. In the absence of a 'mass effect', a small mass, localised peritonitis or haemorrhage should be considered.

Ultrasonography revealed a lobular hypoechoic lesion, roughly 4 cm in diameter, in the mesentery. At laparotomy the mesentery was thickened by a hard, lobular mass, haemorrhage and oedema, and a localised thickening of the jejunum was identified. Histology indicated jejunal lymphoma with local infiltration into the mesentery.

This case illustrates how certain important lesions can produce relatively minor radiographic signs. If these signs are to be recognised, good-quality radiographs must be obtained and interpreted with care.

80 (a) A well-circumscribed, oval soft tissue mass is visible between the bladder and rectum. The ultrasound image shows a hypoechoic, non-cavitated mass which was 2.5 cm in diameter.
(b) In this location, a lesion of the uterine stump is most likely, and the differential diagnosis should include uterine stump granuloma, abscess or neoplasm (Spackman *et al.*, 1984).

The cranial vagina and attached mass were resected. There was no evidence of residual suture material. Histology confirmed pyogranuloma.

81 A single, full-term foetus is present. A soft tissue structure surrounds the foetus, indicating that it is within the uterus. Gas around and within the body of the foetus indicates that it has been dead for a minimum of 6 hours (Farrow, 1976). Gas is also present in the other horn of the uterus.

82 (a) Multiple small gas lucencies overly the urinary bladder and parallel the bladder wall. The prostate is enlarged.
(b) Radiographic diagnosis: emphysematous cystitis compatible with diabetes mellitus and/or infection by gas-forming bacteria.

This dog was diabetic. Emphysematous cystitis (or emphysematous cholecystitis) is occasionally identified in animals with diabetes (Root and Scott, 1971). The gas is produced by bacteria that metabolise glucose in the urine.

83 Several linear filling defects are present in the contrast in the duodenum and jejunum. These have tapered, slightly curved ends. There is no pleating or foreshortening of the affected intestine and no apparent obstruction to contrast passage.

Radiographic diagnosis: ascariasis.

84 (a) A rounded soft tissue mass is present between the os penis and the abdominal wall. No intra-abdominal abnormality is visible.

(b) Differential diagnosis:
- Inguinal mass, e.g. retained testicle, enlarged lymph node.
- Inguinal hernia.

There is no radiographic sign of displacement of abdominal structures, such as the intestine, into this area to support inguinal hernia, hence the most likely diagnosis is inguinal mass. A retained testicle was removed; histology revealed Sertoli-cell tumour.

85 (a) The pneumocystogram shows a thickened cranioventral bladder wall and a focal gas lucency which fills with contrast medium on the double-contrast study, indicating an ulcer or other mucosal defect. Also visible on the double-contrast study is an irregular filling defect adjacent to the mucosal lesion.
(b) Differential diagnosis:
- Ulcerated cystitis.
- Ulcerated neoplasm.
- Urachal diverticulum.
- The filling defect could represent blood clot, inflammatory tissue or neoplasm.

A laparotomy was performed and an ulcerated, thickened portion of the bladder wall with adherent blood clot was resected. The histological diagnosis was chronic ulcerative cystitis.

86 (a) The survey radiograph shows increased opacity and loss of serosal detail in the right cranial quadrant, extending caudally along the right flank. The barium study shows incomplete, irregular filling of the gastric antrum and proximal duodenum. The duodenum has an irregular mucosal pattern and is displaced laterally. These signs indicate infiltration or swelling of the gastric antrum and duodenum associated with a mass effect originating medial to the proximal duodenum. This is the area of the pancreas.
(b) Differential diagnosis:
- Localised enteritis.
- Pancreatitis.
- Other cause of peritonitis, e.g. abdominal abscess.
- Pancreatic neoplasm.
- Other neoplasm, e.g. bile duct carcinoma.

The final diagnosis, based on the clinical and radiographic findings and elevated serum amylase and lipase levels, was pancreatitis (Edwards *et al.*, 1990).

87 (a) The liver is small; there is an oval soft tissue opaque structure between the stomach and transverse large intestine (*Figure 230*, arrows).
(b) Haematology and serum chemistry determinations are indicated to establish whether there is liver dysfunction. The cause of the mass-like lesion caudal to the stomach should be investigated further to determine if it is an intestinal lesion, such as local dilatation, or a mass. Options for further investigation include:
- Additional radiographic projections.
- Upper gastrointestinal barium series.
- Barium enema.
- Ultrasonography.

It was decided to perform an upper gastrointestinal contrast series the following day; however, when a repeat pre-contrast survey radiograph was obtained (*Figure 231*) no sign of the lesion was present. Ultrasonography revealed no abnormality. The dog's clinical condition was much improved after symptomatic treatment and no further investigation was performed. The dog remained well.

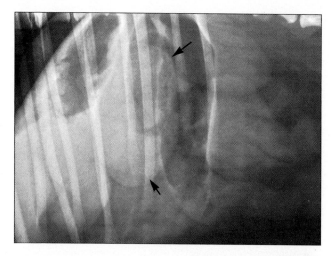

Figure 230

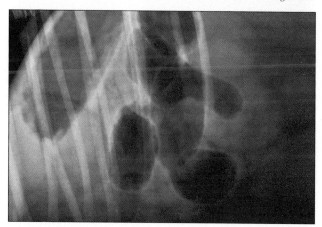

Figure 231

This is an example of an abdominal 'pseudomass', presumably due in this instance to a fortuitous appearance of fluid-filled large intestine. It is not uncommon for superimposed abdominal structures to form a pseudomass, and it is important to examine critically any potential mass to avoid error. In this case, the shape and location were considered atypical for a mass associated with the spleen, pancreas, small intestine or mesentery, suggesting some form of artefact. It is normally a simple matter to repeat radiographs or to perform another diagnostic study if there is any doubt.

88 (a) The bladder is abnormally shaped where the bladder neck joins the urethra; instead of having a smooth, caudally tapered shape, it is blunt. The retrograde urethrogram shows a narrow portion of the proximal urethra.
(b) Radiographic diagnosis: mural lesion at the bladder neck/urethra junction causing partial obstruction of the urethra.

A circumferential urethral mass, 1 cm in diameter, was found at postmortem examination. The histological diagnosis was transitional cell carcinoma (Brearley *et al.*, 1986).

89 (a) The bladder is displaced caudally into the perineal hernia. There is a small volume of vesicoureteral reflux. There is also an incidental finding of lumbosacral disc disease and spondylosis.
(b) The diagnosis is retroflexion of the bladder (White and Herrtage, 1986).

Vesicoureteral reflux is a relatively common finding in dogs undergoing cystography. In many cases it does not represent a significant lesion (Christie, 1973). As in this case, it may occur secondary to displacement of the bladder.

90 (a) An oblong, partially calcified soft tissue mass is seen adjacent to the ventral abdominal wall cranial to the urinary bladder. The mass is not apparently attached to another organ and there is normal serosal detail.
(b) Differential diagnosis:
- Malignant retained testicle.
- Torsion of retained testicle.
- Paraprostatic cyst.
- Peritoneal or mesenteric neoplasm.
- Mesenteric fat necrosis.

A clue to the origin of this mass lies in its shape: testicles have a roughly oblong shape, whereas paraprostatic cysts (and many other masses) tend to be spherical. Repeat physical examination revealed only one scrotal testicle, supporting a diagnosis of retained testicle. The mass was removed at laparotomy. Histology revealed changes compatible with a testicular neoplasm but a definitive diagnosis of tumour type was not possible because of extensive tissue necrosis. The dog's other clinical signs were due to diabetic ketoacidosis.

91 (a) This image is an *operative mesenteric portogram.* It is a positive-contrast study of the portal vein and was obtained by inserting a catheter into a mesenteric vein at laparotomy. Water-soluble organic iodide contrast medium, at a dose of 2 ml/kg body weight, was injected rapidly and a lateral abdominal radiograph was exposed near the end of the injection.
(b) It shows a normal portal vein and its branches to the liver.

Familiarity with the appearance of a normal portogram aids recognition of abnormalities affecting the course or distribution of the portal vein, for example in cases of portosystemic shunting (Schmidt and Suter, 1980).

92 (a) There is a thick tubular viscus in the caudal abdomen. It is clearly thicker than the small intestine, which appears non-distended. Part of this structure overlies the distal large intestine and is directed towards the pelvis.
(b) The radiographic appearance is typical of an enlarged uterus. Differential diagnoses for non-calcified uterine enlargement include early pregnancy, pyometra, mucometra and uterine torsion (rare) (Feeney and Johnston, 1986: Sevelius *et al.*, 1990). In this instance pyometra was confirmed surgically.

93 (a) There are three adjacent structures in the caudal abdomen: the caudal and middle structures are roughly spherical and partially calcified and, although they are together, their outlines are distinct, indicating that they are not in close contact. The caudal structure appears to be continuous with the urethra. The cranial structure is more elongated, with a neck originating from the caudal structure.

(b) From caudal to cranial, these structures are an enlarged prostate, paraprostatic cyst and bladder.

The final diagnosis was benign prostatic hypertrophy with intraprostatic and paraprostatic cysts.

A large paraprostatic cyst may be mistaken for the urinary bladder when the bladder is empty. Cystography is indicated if there is any doubt (White *et al.*, 1987).

94 (a) Pleating (or plication) of the duodenum is visible.

(b) This appearance is characteristic of linear foreign body, such as string or sewing thread.

A piece of cotton thread was removed from the stomach, duodenum and jejunum at laparotomy.

Radiographic findings in cases of linear foreign body include pleating (or plication) of the small intestine, reduced length of affected intestine and peritonitis secondary to enteritis or perforation. The pleating and reduction in length result from peristalsis causing the intestine to 'climb' along the string.

On survey radiographs the intestinal pleating may sometimes be recognised by the presence of a series of eccentric gas bubbles in the affected duodenum and jejunum. On contrast studies the lesion is more visible (Root and Lord, 1971; Felts *et al.*, 1984). Barium clinging to the thread or string produces a thin opaque line which may be visible in the oesophagus and stomach, as it is faintly in this instance (*Figure 232*, arrow).

Figure 232

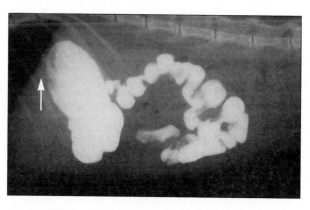

95 There is a focal narrow portion of the contrast column, compatible with an annular thickening of the intestinal wall. The wider, angular shape in the centre of the narrow portion represents an ulcer. This radiographic appearance has been named the 'apple-core sign' of an ulcerated intestinal lesion (Gibbs and Pearson, 1986). The histological diagnosis in this case was adenocarcinoma.

96 (a) The shunt has been partially ligated. Contrast medium is visible in the caudal vena cava (*Figure 233*, dotted arrow) and also in the branches of the hepatic portal veins (small arrows). The liver is small but well vascularised.

(b) The prognosis for this patient is fair to good because the surgery has greatly improved the hepatic portal flow. The prognosis is best when the shunt can be fully occluded without inducing portal hypertension. When portal venous pressure increases after shunt ligation the prognosis is poor because this indicates that the intrahepatic portal veins may be hypoplastic or dysplastic (Johnson *et al.*, 1987).

Figure 233

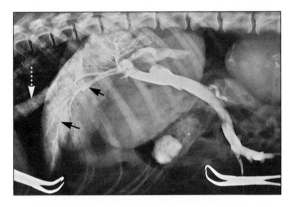

97 (a) There is a consistent focal narrow portion of the distal large intestine and dilatation proximal to it, compatible with an annular thickening of the intestinal wall and partial obstruction.

(b) Large intestinal neoplasm is most likely, although a granulomatous lesion cannot be excluded on the basis of these radiographs.

A large neoplasm with evidence of local spread to regional lymph nodes was confirmed at laparotomy.

If a large intestinal lesion is expected on the basis of clinical signs, barium enema is the radiographic procedure of choice (Biery, 1986); however, as in the case illustrated here, large intestinal lesions may occasionally be identified during an upper gastrointestinal series.

98 A Foley catheter was inserted into the bladder and the cuff inflated with air. Urine was drained out and the bladder inflated with carbon dioxide, producing the negative-contrast cystogram. The distal ureters were opacified by water-soluble organic iodide contrast medium excreted in the urine after intravenous injection. This combination – negative-contrast cystogram and intravenous urogram – normally provides a clear view of the distal ureters and is therefore recommended when investigating lesions such as ectopic ureter.

In this case the position and size of the ureters is normal. Note how the distal ureter curves cranially before inserting in the bladder; loss of this curve and insertion of a caudally directed distal ureter are important signs of ectopia that aid the radiographic diagnosis, particularly when the exact termination of the ureter is not visible (Mason *et al.*, 1990).

99 Both ureters insert at the transition zone between the bladder trigone and cranial urethra, i.e. more caudally than normal. The radiographic diagnosis is bilateral ectopic ureters. Note that the bladder fills with contrast medium despite the abnormal ureter insertion but that the urethra also fills, accounting for the incontinence.

100 (a) The contour of the kidney is distorted by enlargement of the cranial pole. The pelvis is also distorted and there are two rounded, smoothly marginated areas of decreased opacity: a large one in the enlarged cranial pole and a smaller one caudal to it. The relatively lucent appearance of these lesions compared to the remainder of the kidney indicates that they do not contain contrast medium and that, therefore, they may be avascular or cavitary lesions. Similar lesions were visible in the right kidney (not shown).
(b) The presence of multiple, smooth, round, probably cavitary lesions in the kidneys supports a diagnosis of polycystic kidney disease. This was confirmed at postmortem examination.

101 (a) The liver and spleen have similar echogenicity. The surface of the liver has a nodular appearance.
(b) These signs are compatible with a diffuse liver disease causing increased echogenicity and nodularity, for example hepatic cirrhosis. Normally the spleen is more echogenic than the liver, appearing as a lighter shade of grey on the ultrasound image.

Although increased echogenicity and nodularity of the liver are typical of cirrhosis, many ultrasonographic findings in the liver and spleen are non-specific and biopsy is usually required to confirm a diagnosis (Lamb, 1991b).

102 Differential diagnoses for hypoechoic hepatic lesions:
- Primary hepatic neoplasm.
- Metastasis.
- Lymphoma.
- Hepatic nodular hyperplasia.
- Hepatitis.
- Cyst.
- Abscess.
- Haematoma.

103 ● Chronic inflammation, i.e. cholecystitis.
  ● Cystic mucinous hyperplasia, an age-related change.
Other causes reported in humans include hepatic cirrhosis, acute viral hepatitis, congestive heart failure, hypoalbuminaemia, renal failure and ascites (Wegener *et al.*, 1987).

104 (a) There is a focal, round, non-encapsulated hypoechoic lesion.
(b) It represents some form of nodule. Lymphoma is a common cause of this type of lesion in the spleen and liver; however, this finding is non-specific because lymphoid hyperplasia, early primary neoplasm and metastasis can also produce hypoechoic nodules in the spleen (Lamb *et al.*, 1991a).

105   *Figure 234.* There is a *mirror-image* artefact producing a spurious image of the liver (M) on the left, apparently cranial to the line of the diaphragm. An artefactual split in the diaphragm is visible (arrow), caused by *refraction* of the ultrasound beam passing through the cranial aspect of the liver (Middleton and Melson, 1988).

Figure 234

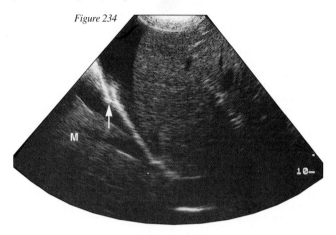

106   (a) The abnormalities are:
- Loss of clarity of the internal architecture of the kidney associated with increased echogenicity of the medulla.
- Mild dilatation of the renal pelvis, i.e. hydronephrosis.

(b) Differential diagnosis:
- Chronic nephritis, e.g. pyelonephritis, feline infectious peritonitis.
- Lymphoma.

Note that the hydronephrosis is not necessarily a sign of urinary obstruction; it is commonly seen when infiltrative or fibrotic diseases of the kidney cause distortion of the parenchyma which pulls the pelvis out of shape. In this case the final diagnosis was lymphoma (Walter *et al.*, 1988).

107   There is a hypoechoic mass, approximately 2.5 cm, in diameter with a gas-filled centre. Artefacts associated with the gas obscure the far wall of the mass, producing a horseshoe-shaped appearance. The mass is caused by a focal thickening of the intestinal wall; the gas represents the intestinal lumen. (Note that this is a transverse image of the intestine; twisting the transducer through 90° would produce a longitudinal image showing a length of affected intestine.)

This appearance is typical of neoplasia, although granulomatous lesions can produce similar signs. In cats, adenocarcinoma and lymphoma commonly account for such lesions (Nyland and Kantrowitz, 1986). Histology in this instance indicated lymphoma.

108   (a) A highly echogenic structure, approximately 2 cm in diameter, is producing an acoustic shadow which obscures the bladder wall beyond the lesion.

(b) This is a urinary calculus.

Acoustic shadowing beyond a lesion on an ultrasound scan results from attenuation of the beam by the lesion. It is often associated with calcified lesions (Kremkau and Taylor, 1986).

Musculoskeletal System

109 (a) The condyles fuse together at about 6 weeks and fuse to the distal humerus at 6–8 months.
(b) 8–12 months.
(c) 16–24 weeks.
(d) The tibial tuberosity fuses with the tibial condyles at 6–8 months, and with the tibial crest at 6–12 months (Ticer, 1984).

110 (a) Dorsoplantar – provides an unsuperimposed view of the medial trochlear ridge, the most common site of the lesion.
(b) Flexed mediolateral – flexed to avoid superimposition by the anconeal process by the medial epicondyle of the humerus.
(c) Ventrodorsal; however, if a luxation is not apparent, a lateral view should be obtained. Only when both views are normal can one reliably state that the joint is not luxated.
(d) Dorsoventral – provides a view of both zygomatic arches projected well away from the cranium.

111
● Over-exposure – too high kVp, mAs, short film–focus distance or wrong film–screen system.
● Over-development – film left in developer tank too long, or temperature of solution too high.
● Film fogged by light – inappropriate safe light in darkroom or leakage of light into darkroom or damaged cassette.

112
● There are only 6 lumbar vertebrae.
● There is dorsal displacement of the caudal sacral end-plate, i.e. a Salter type 1 physeal fracture.
It is important to approach any radiograph in a methodical manner. For example, examining the peripheral parts of the image and looking at basic anatomical details such as the number of vertebrae (or toes, teeth, etc) aids identification of abnormalities.

113 Poorly circumscribed foci of increased opacity are visible, affecting the diaphysis of the left femur (*Figure 235*, arrow). This appearance is characteristic of panosteitis.
Panosteitis is a common problem in young dogs, producing non-specific signs of ill health and painful bones. Direct palpation of an affected bone is necessary to locate the source of pain. In many cases the diagnosis is made radiographically; however, the lesions are not always apparent in the early stages of the disease, and repeat studies at intervals of 2–4-weeks may be necessary before the diagnosis can be confirmed (Bohning *et al.*, 1970).

114 There is an oblique fracture of the right femoral neck (*Figure 236*, dotted arrow) and a minimally displaced physeal fracture of the left femoral head, visible as a step (arrow) at the physis.
If you missed one of these lesions, try to remember that the effects of trauma are unpredictable and that multiple injuries are common. Therefore, when evaluating radiographs of trauma cases make sure you look for the second (and third) lesion (Daly, 1978).

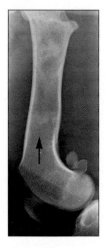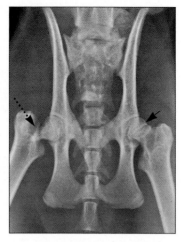

Figure 235   *Figure 236*

115 (a) The lesion is characterised by:
- Prominent collars of calcification surrounding the metaphyses.
- Sclerotic metaphyses.
- Soft tissue swelling.

(b) This is metaphyseal osteopathy (*synonym*: hypertrophic osteodystrophy).

At earlier stages of the disease, radiographs may show soft-tissue swelling and a characteristic lucent line traversing the distal radius and ulnar metaphyses parallel to the growth plates. Subsequent calcification of the swelling produces the large, often dramatic, perimetaphyseal collars seen in this instance (Grondalen, 1976).

Diagnosis is usually straightforward because the radiographic signs are characteristic of this condition. However, the aetiology and pathogenesis are not established (Woodard, 1982). Recent work implicates distemper virus infection (Mee *et al.*, 1992) and it is interesting to speculate that the systemic signs in this animal were associated with distemper. This dog was destroyed because of its severe, unremitting pain, anorexia and continued systemic signs.

116 (a) Both coxofemoral joints are subluxated, and periarticular osteophytes are present, indicating arthrosis. The gluteal muscles are small, compatible with muscle wasting secondary to reduced activity.

(b) These changes are diagnostic of hip dysplasia (Lust *et al.*, 1985).

117 (a) There are several lesions:
- The L2/3 intervertebral disc space is narrow, and opaque material overlies the spinal canal at this level.
- The L4/5 intervertebral disc space is narrow.
- Partial calcification of intervertebral discs at T13/L1, L4/5 and L5/6.
- There are only 6 lumbar vertebrae.
- Transitional lumbosacral vertebra.

(b) The dog's clinical signs are compatible with a spinal cord injury cranial to L3; the calcified disc prolapse at L2/3 is most likely to be the cause. Although there is radiographic evidence of disc prolapse at L4/5, this would be expected to reduce hindlimb muscle tone and to reduce patellar reflexes, i.e. a lower motor neurone lesion. Sites of calcified, non-displaced intervertebral discs represent potential sites of disc prolapse. The finding of 6 lumbar vertebrae and the transitional lumbosacral vertebra are unlikely to be significant.

The clinical signs in this case were relatively mild, and conservative medical treatment was adopted. A myelogram was not performed; however, had the dog's condition deteriorated and surgical treatment become necessary, a myelogram would be recommended in order to confirm the site of cord injury and to guide the surgical approach.

118 There is:
- Luxation of the patella.
- A fractured canine tooth fragment adjacent to the tibial crest.
- Extensive emphysema.

Overlapping of the patella and distal femur on this view indicates luxation; a craniocaudal (or caudocranial) view is required to determine whether it is luxated medially or laterally.

Tooth fragments are occasionally found in fight wounds in dogs and cats. They may be distinguished from fragments of fractured bone by their characteristic shape, lack of trabecular pattern and greater opacity than cortical bone. In some instances additional radiographs may be required to locate a tooth fragment accurately prior to attempted removal.

119 (a) There is remodelling of the plantar aspect of the fibular tarsal bone (*Figure 237*, arrow) compatible with enthesopathy of the plantar ligament attachments, and soft tissue swelling on the plantar aspect compatible with a plantar ligament injury.
(b) A dorsoplantar view is indicated to provide an additional view of the tarsal joints. Also, a hyperextended (stressed) lateral radiograph (*Figure 238*) is indicated to evaluate instability associated with the plantar ligament lesion. In this instance it reveals marked intertarsal subluxation.

This example illustrates the value of obtaining stressed radiographs in cases with suspected joint instability (Farrow, 1982).

120 ● Joint effusion.
- Periarticular osteophytes (many cases have pre-existing joint disease).
- Small bone fragment adjacent to the tibial plateau due to avulsion of cruciate ligament insertion.
- Subluxation due to cranial displacement of the tibia (uncommon).

121 ● Panosteitis.
- Osseous metastasis.
- Hypertrophic osteopathy ('Marie's disease').

122 ● Metaphyseal osteopathy (*synonym*: hypertrophic osteodystrophy).
- Retained cartilage core in the ulna.
- Primary bone tumour.
- Lead poisoning (rare).
- Rickets (rare).

123 ●Thyroid carcinoma.
- Mammary carcinoma.
- Prostate carcinoma.
- Haemangiosarcoma.
  (Russel and Walker, 1983.)

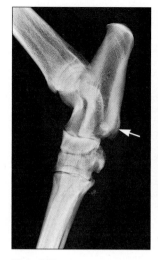 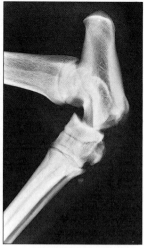

Figure 237 *Figure 238*

124 There is subluxation of the humeroradial and humeroulnar joints and a medial condyle fracture. The fracture line passes through the epiphysis, physis and medial metaphysis. This physeal fracture may be classified as Salter–Harris type IV (Brinkner *et al.*, 1990). In this animal there is an additional small bone fragment adjacent to the medial coronoid process on the craniocaudal view, which could represent an additional articular fracture or medial collateral ligament avulsion.

125 (a) Stifle arthrosis is present, characterised by:
- Prominent periarticular osteophytes.
- Joint effusion.
- Flattened, irregular subchondral plate on the lateral femoral condyle (*Figure 239*, arrow).

  (b) Differential diagnosis:
- Primary degenerative joint disease.
- Degenerative joint disease secondary to osteochondrosis, cruciate ligament injury, or other chronic joint injury.
- Bacterial arthritis.

The flattened subchondral plate on the lateral femoral condyle is a characteristic sign of osteochondrosis (Poulos, 1982).

Many cases of osteochondrosis develop clinical signs within the first 6 months of life, and this usually leads to diagnosis at an early age. In some animals the resulting lameness is sufficiently mild or intermittent for the owner to seek no advice until the secondary changes are advanced, as in this instance.

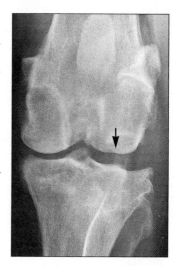

Figure 239

126 The radiograph (*Figure 126*) shows loss of bone protuberances along the entire medial aspect of the limb, affecting the medial malleolus, medial aspect of the the talus including the trochlear ridge, central tarsal bone, proximal and distal second metacarpal and first phalanx. The first and second tarsal bones are lost. Less evident on the radiograph is extensive loss of soft tissues covering the medial aspect.

This is an abrasion injury. It occurs during car accidents when part of the body (typically the tarsus) is rubbed forcibly along the surface of the road. The usual result is extensive soft tissue and bone loss which leaves affected joints open, unstable and contaminated (Aron, 1988).

127 There is a comminuted fracture of the first phalanx, second digit (*Figure 240*, large arrow). Note that the lesion is not visible on the lateral view and that on a dorsoplantar view the edges of the pads produce potentially confusing lines (small arrows), that could mimic phalangeal fractures.

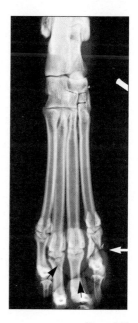

Figure 240

149

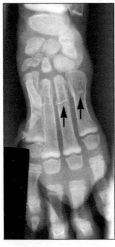

128 (a) Transverse fractures of the right fourth and fifth metacarpals are visible (*Figure 241,* arrows). Both paws are osteopenic, with thin cortices and relatively opaque metaphyses; these are seen best at the distal radius and distal metacarpals.
(b) Radiographic diagnosis: pathological metacarpal fractures secondary to osteopenia, probably of nutritional origin, e.g. nutritional secondary hyperparathyroidism.
(c) Treatment is two-fold: support the fractures and improve the diet.

Figure 241

129 (a) There is an aggressive-appearing lesion partially destroying the shaft of the fourth metatarsal. The bone is expanded, the cortex is thin and there is a spiculated periosteal reaction. A wire is embedded in the pad adjacent to the bone lesion, and the soft tissues of the paw are swollen.
(b) Differential diagnosis:
   ● Osteomyelitis, possibly associated with the foreign body.
   ● Primary bone tumour.
The most likely diagnosis in this case is influenced by geographical location. For example, in parts of North America (such as the Mississippi and Ohio river valleys or southern California) fungal osteomyelitis due to *Blastomyces* or *Coccidioides* could produce this lesion (Ackerman and Spencer, 1982), in which case the wire might be the portal of entry of the organism. In Europe, fungal osteomyelitis is rare so primary bone tumour would be more likely.
   The histological diagnosis in this case was osteosarcoma. (The wire was an incidental finding).

130 (a) This is a special projection designed to provide an unsuperimposed view of the dorsal acetabular rim. To achieve this the dog is positioned in sternal recumbency with the hindlimbs extended cranially and the paws elevated. This position tilts the pelvis so that a vertical X-ray beam passes along its long axis. This view may be described as a craniodorsal–caudoventral oblique.
(b) There is a chip fracture of the right dorsal acetabular rim. The irregular rounded appearance of the fracture edges indicates an injury of at least months' duration; the fracture line is still visible, indicating a non-union.

150

The dorsal acetabular rim radiographic view was devised to aid the preoperative assessment of hip dysplasia (Slocum and Devine, 1990). In this case it was obtained to provide an alternative view of the dorsal acetabular rim lesion, which was suspected but not seen clearly on the ventrodorsal view.

131 (a) Periarticular osteophytes are visible on the anconeal process (*Figure 242*, dotted arrow) and overlying the margins of the semilunar notch of the ulna, producing a sclerotic appearance on the mediolateral view (arrow). The craniocaudal view is slightly oblique to show the craniomedial aspect and demonstrates a smooth, round bone fragment adjacent to the humeroulnar joint (*Figure 243*, arrow).
(b) Radiographic diagnosis: elbow arthrosis secondary to fragmented medial coronoid process (Olsson, 1983).

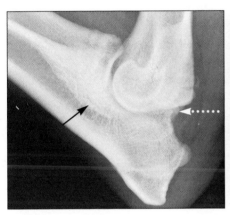 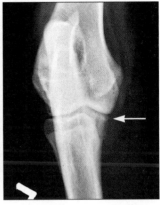

Figure 242   *Figure 243*

132 (a) Definition of the joint margins has been lost due to widespread, indistinct, and therefore active-appearing, periarticular osteophytes which extend along the metaphyses. There is irregularity of the subchondral plate on the femoral and tibial condyles, subchondral sclerosis affecting the medial aspect of the tibial plateau and sclerosis under the washer. Finally, there is a sharply marginated area of bone resorption on the lateral aspect of the distal femur and soft tissue swelling.
(b) The severity of these changes, and particularly the subchondral erosions, supports a diagnosis of bacterial arthritis, probably secondary to surgery and exacerbated by the presence of synthetic material in the joint.
(c) Joint fluid aspirate will provide a sample for cytology and culture to confirm the diagnosis. In this instance a large volume of blood-stained cloudy fluid containing large numbers of polymorph neutrophils and bacteria was obtained.
    The joint was re-explored and the implants removed. A subtotal synovectomy was performed and the dog was given a course of amoxycillin. The lameness was greatly reduced 1 month later.

133 Calcified lesions associated with joints:
- Calcified cartilage flap due to osteochondrosis.
- Calcifying tendinopathy.
- Avulsion fracture of tendon or ligament insertion.
- Articular fracture.
- Calcified synovial membrane lesion, e.g. synovial osteochondrometaplasia, dystrophic calcification secondary to corticosteroid injection.
- Calcinosis circumscripta (*synonym*: tumoral calcinosis).
- Intrameniscal calcification in cats.
- Ununited anconeal process.

134 Advantages of the cisterna magna route include:
- Generally easier to place the needle.
- Ability to collect an adequate cerebrospinal fluid sample.
- Unlikely to produce epidural deposition of contrast medium.

Advantages of the lumbar route include:
- More likely to achieve immediate distribution of contrast medium throughout the length of the vertebral canal.
- More likely to deposit contrast both cranial and caudal to a space-occupying lesion and, therefore, more likely to show its full extent.

135 Indications for myelography:
- To identify a suspected spinal lesion not visible on survey radiographs.
- To evaluate a known spinal lesion that does not correlate with the clinical signs.
- To determine the extent of a survey radiographic lesion.
- To help to plan the surgical approach to a spinal lesion.

136
- Extradural, i.e. originating outside the dura.
- Intradural–extramedullary, i.e. originating between the dura and the spinal cord.
- Intramedullary, i.e. originating within the spinal cord.

137
- Blood vessel, e.g. the vertebral artery at the level of C2 is normally visible passing through the subarachnoid space ventral to the spinal cord.
- Intradural neoplasm, e.g. neurofibroma.
- Air bubble, introduced during myelography.

138 (a) There is an extradural lesion at the level of the C6/7 intervertebral disc space displacing the dura and spinal cord dorsally. The spinal cord is narrow at this point, indicating that the lesion causes compression.
(b) When traction is applied the lesion is reduced. This indicates that the lesion is dynamic (i.e. it changes with changes in body position), and therefore it is *flexible*. Thickened connective tissue structures (i.e. the dorsal longitudinal ligament and/or dorsal annulus fibrosus) are usually responsible for these lesions (Seim and Withrow, 1982). In this case, a markedly thickened annulus fibrosus was identified at surgery.

139 (a) The vertebrae, ribs and sternebrae are diffusely sclerotic with loss of the normal trabecular pattern, producing a chalk-like appearance.
(b) This indicates osteopetrosis, an occasional finding in old cats. The pathogenesis of this condition is not established (Kramers *et al.*, 1988).

140 (a) A moderately well-defined lucent zone is visible in the rostral mandible adjacent to the incisor tooth roots. The incisors are malaligned. The lamina dura surrounding most of the incisor roots is preserved, but it is absent on the lingual aspect of the left canine.

(b) Differential diagnoses:
- Inflammatory gingival lesion eroding bone.
- Tooth root abscess.
- Soft tissue neoplasm invading bone, e.g. squamous cell carcinoma.
- Epulis.
- Primary bone tumour, e.g. fibrosarcoma.

Histology revealed proliferative epithelial cells invading the adjacent bone. The diagnosis was acanthomatous epulis. Of the three categories of epulis (fibrous, ossifying and acanthomatous), acanthomatous is most often associated with invasion of the underlying bone.

The epulides have recently been reclassified as neoplasms (Bostok and White, 1987).

141 (a) Bone scintigraphy is performed by intravenous injection of a radiochemical that becomes attached to bone. ^{99m}Tc-methylene diphosphonate is normally used. After a delay of about 3 hours, images are acquired using a Gamma camera. By this time, most of the radionuclide is incorporated into bone, and the result is an image of the skeleton. Typically, each image is composed of 100,000–250,000 counts and can be viewed on a monitor screen or printed onto photographic paper or radiographic film as a permanent record.

The highest rates of radionuclide uptake, which appear as dark areas on the scintigraphic image, correspond to areas of rapid bone metabolism such as growth plates or active bone lesions. Bone scintigraphy represents a sensitive method of surveying the skeleton for lesions that may be invisible on radiographs (Lamb, 1991a).

(b) Multiple foci of increased radionuclide uptake are visible, mainly affecting the ribs and sternum. This appearance is characteristic of osseous metastasis.

The diagnosis in this animal was metastatic prostatic carcinoma.

142 (a) There is cranial luxation of the right coxofemoral joint. Also there is asymmetry of the sacroiliac joints: the left appears relatively normal but the right involves part of the lateral process of the seventh lumbar vertebra.

(b) The right femoral neck is narrow and the head is small and osteopenic compared with the left. These signs indicate bone remodelling secondary to the luxation which, therefore, must be several weeks old.

Radiographic diagnosis: chronic right coxofemoral luxation; asymmetrical pelvic attachment to the spine.

The owner later admitted that the cat had shown signs of an injury to its right hindlimb 5 weeks before it was brought for examination. It may be assumed that the luxation occurred then.

The significance of asymmetrical pelvic attachment in this case is uncertain; however, asymmetrical pelvic attachment in dogs is sometimes associated with unilateral hip dysplasia (Morgan and Rosenblatt, 1987). It is conceivable that it in some way acted as a predisposing factor in this animal.

143 (a) Radiographic abnormalities include:
- Local increased opacity of the caudal part of the body of the fourth lumbar vertebra.
- Apparent bone fragment overlying the intervertebral foramen on the lateral view.
- Wedge-shaped L4/5 intervertebral disc space on the ventrodorsal view.
- Displacement of the caudal end-plate of the fourth lumbar vertebra also on the ventrodorsal view.

(b) Compression fracture of the fourth lumbar vertebra.

The cat's condition did not improve and it was destroyed 2 days later.

The radiographic signs associated with minimally displaced fractures are often subtle and necessitate high-quality radiographs and careful interpretation. The wedge-shaped intevertebral disc space in this case may also indicate traumatic disc prolapse; however, this would require a myelogram for confirmation (McKee, 1990; Selcer *et al.*, 1991).

144 (a) There is carpal joint disease characterised by large, well-defined periarticular osteophytes, loss of definition of the intercarpal and carpometacarpal joints and soft tissue swelling.

(b) The radiographs indicate chronic carpal arthrosis. There is no radiographic sign that specifically indicates bacterial arthritis or other aggressive aetiology.

Synovial fluid analysis indicated non-septic inflammation and a Coombs test was negative. Final diagnosis: acute exacerbation of chronic arthrosis.

It is not uncommon for dogs with long-standing arthrosis to suffer acute exacerbation of signs and to present with such a sore joint that some other more serious cause is suspected. In these animals, radiographs usually show advanced bone lesions which reflect the chronicity of the underlying condition *not* the cause of the acute pain. The diagnosis of more aggressive aetiologies such as immune-mediated bacterial arthritis or joint neoplasm should be supported by synovial fluid analysis and/or synovial biopsy (Allen, 1986).

145 ● Salter–Harris type II fracture of the proximal tibia.

● Segmental fracture of the fibula.

The tibial fracture was reduced surgically and stabilised using crossed pins. Healing was uneventful and the pins were removed 5 weeks later (Brinkner *et al.*, 1990).

146 (a) There are oblique fractures of the mid-diaphyses of the radius and ulna, with moderate cranial displacement of the distal portion of the limb.

(b) *Figure 150* shows:

● Malunion due to angulation.

● Humeroulnar subluxation.

● Premature distal ulnar growth plate closure.

The humeroulnar subluxation is caused by asynchronous growth between the radius and ulna. In this case, it is probably due to a combination of synostosis at the fracture site *and* damage to the distal ulnar growth plate associated with the original injury.

Angular limb deformities and/or elbow lesions commonly occur secondary to forelimb injuries in puppies. The potential for complications, particularly those associated with distal radial or ulnar growth plate injuries, should be remembered when the acute injury is evaluated (Shields-Henney and Gambardella, 1989; Brinker *et al.*, 1990).

147 (a) Amorphous calcification surrounds the right coxofemoral joint. Associated bone lesions are present, including subluxation, remodelling of the medial aspect of the acetabulum and femoral neck, and delayed closure of the femoral head physis. A small calcified lesion is present adjacent to the left greater trochanter.

(b) Radiographic diagnosis: joint-associated calcification inducing secondary bone changes, possibly due to pressure.

Histological examination of a biopsy showed calcinosis circumscripta (*synonym*: tumoral calcinosis). This is an idiopathic sporadic condition producing calcified masses, usually in the skin (Scott and Buerger, 1988) or close to joints, including the coxofemoral joint. There is a breed predisposition for German shepherd dogs. These lesions do not usually cause signs of pain or dysfunction (Marks *et al.*, 1991).

Another diagnosis that might be considered on the basis of this radiograph is synovial chondrometaplasia (Flo *et al.*, 1987).

148 (a) On the lateral view (*Figure 153*) there is a prominent irregular exostosis with an opaque edge arising on the ventral aspect of the mandible. The ventrodorsal (intraoral) view (*Figure 154*) shows a massive, solid-appearing exostosis along the medial aspect of the right mandibular ramus, which is approximately twice normal thickness. The size and appearance of the lesion indicate a chronic, non-aggressive aetiology.
(b) Craniomandibular osteopathy (Riser *et al.*, 1967).

149 This oblique distal tibia fracture has occurred through an abnormally thin part of the cortex. The metaphysis is lucent and normal trabecular pattern absent. Therefore, this is a pathological fracture secondary to a bone-destroying lesion and the fracture is not repairable. The limb was amputated. The histological diagnosis was osteosarcoma.

A pathological fracture should be suspected following an acute fracture whenever the bone edges are thin or indistinct and local osteopenia is identified. Remember that many primary bone tumours affect the metaphysis of a long bone and that they may occur in young animals (Quigley and Leedale, 1983; Phillips *et al.*, 1986).

150 (a) There is a diffuse irregular periosteal reaction affecting the entire diaphysis. The bone has a stippled opacity due to the overlying periosteal reaction and possibly because of focal lucencies within the cortex. This appearance supports an aggressive aetiology but the diaphyseal location is atypical for a primary bone tumour.
(b) Differential diagnoses:
- Metastasis, e.g. from mammary neoplasm.
- Non-osseous primary tumour, e.g. haemangiosarcoma.
- Osteomyelitis.

Biopsy revealed haemangiosarcoma.

A large number of primary bone sarcomas are described in animals (Moulton, 1990). Osteosarcoma, fibrosarcoma and chondrosarcoma are the most common types; however, other cell types not specific for bone may give rise to neoplasms (including haemangiosarcoma, lymphoma, myeloma, reticulum cell sarcoma and liposarcoma). As in this animal, the radiographic appearance of the less common types is often different from that associated with osteo/fibro/chondrosarcoma (Moulton, 1990).

151 (a) An ill-defined, poorly circumscibed lucency affects the proximal metaphysis of the radius; it extends distally to the mid-diaphysis and includes focal areas of cortical lucency and faint periosteal response. There is no sign of elbow arthrosis.
(b) The radiographic lesion is not centred on the elbow. It is an aggressive bone lesion originating in the radial metaphysis and, therefore, primary bone tumour is the principal differential diagnosis. Biopsy confirmed osteosarcoma.

The classic radiographic signs of primary bone tumour (85% of which are osteosarcomas), such as a florid 'sunburst' periosteal response, are seen only in a small proportion of cases.

Many osteosarcomas produce more modest radiographic lesions, which nevertheless have signs of aggressive biological behaviour including ill-defined margins, bone lysis and pathological fracture (Ling *et al.*, 1974; Gibbs *et al.*, 1984).

152 (a) There is deformity of the distal diaphysis and metaphysis of the femur, characterised by a smoothly marginated increase in width and opacity of the bone, with preservation of most of the trabecular pattern. Lucent lines with sclerotic margins traverse the bone. The distal femoral physis is closed.
(b) This is a malunion. The location and shape of callus suppport a Salter type II fracture with a large metaphyseal component. The relatively normal alignment indicates that the fracture was minimally displaced (Nunamaker *et al.*, 1985).

153 (a) Flattening and irregularity of the subchondral plate is visible on the caudal aspect of both humeral heads (*Figures 244* and *245*, arrows). This appearance is pathognomonic for osteochondrosis. A small, faintly calcified lesion is adjacent to the caudal edge of the left humeral head (*Figure 245*, dotted arrow). This may represent a calcified detached cartilage flap, i.e. osteochondrosis *dissecans*.
(b) The arthrograms (*Figures 246* and *247*) show a large flap of loose cartilage attached to the right humerus (arrow) but there is no attached flap remaining on the left. The presence of a loose flap has been correlated with lameness (van Bree *et al.*, 1992) and the arthrograms explain why the dog has pain in its right shoulder but not in the left. Arthrotomy of the right shoulder was performed and the loose flap removed.

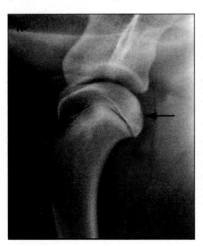

Figure 244

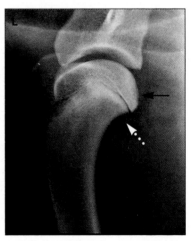

Figure 245

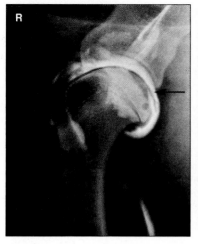
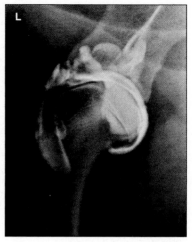

Figure 246   Figure 247

154 (a) The right femoral head is small, mis-shapen and osteopenic compared with the left. The dorsal aspect of the femoral head is flattened and there is a narrow lucency paralleling the subchondral plate. The right femoral neck is thicker than the left and has exostoses compatible with capsular osteophytes. The right femur is short. Also, there is reduced muscle mass on the right.
(b) Radiographic diagnosis: ischaemic necrosis of the right femoral head (*synonym*: Legg–Calvé–Perthes disease) (Lee, 1974).

155 There is extensive gas in the subcutaneous tissues. A poorly defined structure is seen caudal to the distal femur, producing a laminated-appearing opacity close to that of the surrounding tissues. This represents a wooden foreign body. No fracture is visible.
   Many wooden foreign bodies are difficult to identify radiographically because they are small and have a similar opacity to soft tissues (Mucci and Stenhouse, 1985; Kerr and Kirker-Head, 1989). Hence wood is most likely to be recognised when it is large and/or located in a thin part of the body which can provide a high-quality radiograph with minimal scattered radiation. In this case the wood fragment was removed surgically and the surrounding tissues debrided and flushed. The wound healed uneventfully.

156 (a) There is destruction of the dorsal part of the cranial end-plate of the third cervical vertebra. There is no apparent bone production associated with this lesion. It is visible on both views.

157

(b) Radiographic diagnosis: bone tumour, probably primary.

Without well-positioned and carefully interpreted radiographs, a small lesion such as this could easily be missed. However, despite its size, the radiological features of this lesion – localised, poorly marginated, predominantly osteolytic – are typical of primary vertebral neoplasms (Morgan *et al.*, 1980). Thoracic radiographs obtained after detection of the spine lesion revealed multiple pulmonary nodules. The final diagnosis was primary undifferentiated sarcoma of the spine with lung metastasis.

157 (a) Mild intramedullary swelling, centred at T12/13 (and the T12/13 intervertebral disc space is narrow).

(b) Radiographic diagnosis: spinal cord oedema secondary to intervertebral disc prolapse at T12/13.

The clinical signs in this case were considered severe enough to warrant surgical treatment. Therefore, the myelogram was performed to confirm the site of the lesion, to rule out other potential problems and to give the surgeon a guide to whether the prolapse was asymmetrical (and a candidate for hemilaminectomy).

It is not uncommon for dogs with acute signs of disc prolapse to show myelographic evidence of spinal cord swelling due to oedema. The more chronic a disc prolapse is, the less likely it is to be associated with cord swelling and the more likely it is to produce the classic extradural sign on a myelogram.

In this animal a left-sided hemilaminectomy was performed, confirming disc prolapse at T12/13 and revealing extensive subdural haemorrhage. The dog showed gradual improvement after surgery, emptying its bladder normally after 4 days and standing unaided after 6 days.

158 (a) There is an extradural lesion at the level of L1. It displaces the spinal cord slightly ventrally and to the left.

(b) Differential diagnoses:
- Extradural neoplasm, e.g. lymphoma, haemangiosarcoma, lipoma.
- Inflammatory extradural lesion, e.g. due to migrating foreign body.
- Haematoma.
- Atypical intervertebral disc prolapse.

A bone tumour such as osteosarcoma or metastasis was considered unlikely in the absence of a radiographic bone lesion. A hemilaminectomy was performed and an extradural mass was partially removed. Histology indicated lymphoma (Gilmore, 1983; Dallman and Sanders, 1986).

159 (a) This lesion is characterised by:
- Predominantly osteoblastic reaction affecting the bodies and lateral processes of L2–L4.
- Ventral soft tissue swelling.
- No apparent involvement of the intervertebral disc spaces, end-plates or dorsal laminae.

(b) Differential diagnosis:
- Chronic osteomyelitis.
- Secondary neoplasia (less likely).
- Hepatozoonosis (principally in the tropics).

The fact that this lesion affects three adjacent vertebrae to the same degree makes chronic osteomyelitis the principal differential diagnosis in this animal.

Primary neoplasia would affect one bone predominantly, if not exclusively. Secondary neoplasia, i.e. tumour invading the spine either by direct extension from a primary in the retroperitoneum or via the vertebral venous sinuses, is plausible. Prostatic carcinoma frequently spreads to the lumbar spine in this way, but invariably affects the caudal lumbar vertebrae.

It is thought that the mid-lumbar spine is predisposed to infection by migrating foreign bodies, such as grass awns, which travel from the intestine into the mesentery and from there to the retroperitoneum immediately ventral to L3/4 (Johnston and Summers, 1971). *Nocardia* spp. are sometimes involved in this site (Mitten, 1974). Biopsy confirmed osteomyelitis.

160 There is destruction of the caudal aspect of L7, right side of the sacrum and right ilium. The margins of the lesion have no apparent sclerosis, indicating a highly aggressive bone-destroying process. The involvement of three adjacent bones indicates that the lesion is not confined by joints and that it is probably not a primary bone neoplasm (Morgan *et al.*, 1980).

Radiographic diagnosis: soft tissue neoplasm, possibly of joint or nerve origin, invading bone.

The histological diagnosis was spindle-cell sarcoma; the exact tissue of origin could not be established.

161 (a) There is marked swelling of the toe and partial destruction of the third phalanx, which is ill-defined and decalcified compared with the other toes. This indicates an aggressive aetiology, such as nail-bed neoplasm, although an aggressive bacterial or fungal infection could also produce these signs. The thoracic radiographs show a soft tissue mass in the right caudal lung lobe.

(b) The radiographic signs are compatible with nail-bed neoplasia with solitary metastasis to the lung. However, it is not usual for metastasis to produce a single large lung lesion, hence a primary lung neoplasm, granuloma or other lesion cannot be excluded on the basis of these radiographs. Biopsy of both sites indicated sweat-gland carcinoma, i.e. primary skin neoplasm with metastasis to the lung.

Malignant neoplasia of the nail bed in cats may affect single or multiple toes; metastasis to lung and bone has been reported (Ackerman and Spencer, 1985).

In certain parts of the world, fungal infections of the nail beds are more common than neoplasia. Radiography cannot reliably distinguish these aetiologies, and histology and/or fungal culture is required.

162 (a) On the survey radiographs the dorsal lamina of T12 is thickened and sclerotic and the dorsal border of the vertebral body is concave. The myelogram shows ventral displacement and narrowing of the spinal cord (i.e. compression) secondary to the dorsal lamina lesion.

(b) The radiographic findings of focal osteoblastic bone lesion and remodelling of the ventral floor of the vertebral canal indicate a *gradually* enlarging lesion. An aggressive aetiology is unlikely, hence the differential diagnosis should include:

● Low-grade inflammatory bone lesion, i.e. chronic osteomyelitis.

● Slow-growing osteoblastic neoplasm, e.g. osteochondroma (*synonym*: ossifying cartilagenous exostosis) (Reiderson *et al.,* 1988).

● Fracture callus.

The entire affected portion of T12 was removed at laminectomy. The cat made a steady recovery and regained normal hindlimb function. The histological diagnosis was fracture callus.

Head and Neck

163 (a) 3142/3143.
(b) 3131/3121.

164 7 months.

165 There is a stone in the nasopharynx.
The stone was removed orally after retracting the soft palate. It was too large to enter the nasopharynx via the nose, hence it must have been coughed into the nasopharynx from the pharynx.

166 There are areas of increased soft tissue/fluid opacity affecting the left and, to a lesser extent, the right nasal chambers. Also on the left are two well-demarcated focal lucencies (*Figure 248*, arrows). The turbinates are not visible on the left or mid-right nasal chambers. The vomer bone (arrowheads) is unaffected, despite this being a bilateral lesion.

Radiographic diagnosis: aggressive nasal disease. The principal differential diagnoses are fungal rhinitis and primary nasal tumour. The presence of well-defined focal lucencies has been correlated with aspergillosis. This dog is too young for any primary nasal tumour except lymphoma. Aspergillosis was confirmed by serology and culture of nasal washings (Harvey *et al.*, 1979; Sullivan *et al.*, 1986).

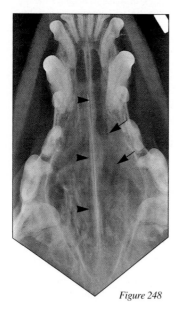

Figure 248

167   There is soft tissue/fluid opacity throughout the right nasal chamber; turbinate detail is obliterated, producing a relatively homogeneous appearance. The vomer appears slightly eroded on the right side (*Figure 249*, arrowhead) and is displaced to the left at the level of the second premolars. There is calculus on the canine teeth (arrows).

Radiographic diagnosis: aggressive lesion arising in the right nasal chamber, compatible with primary neoplasia.

Adenocarcinoma was confirmed by histology (Harvey *et al.*, 1979; Sullivan *et al.*, 1987).

Figure 249

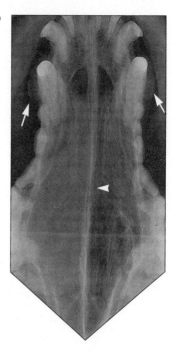

168   (a) The left external ear canal is not visible (the right is indicated on *Figure 250* by the arrow), probably because of blockage by exudate or tissue swelling. The left tympanic bulla is more opaque than the right, compatible with fluid and/or soft tissue content, and the bone is slightly thicker.

(b) Radiographic diagnosis: chronic otitis media.

The regular thickening of the left bulla is typical of the response of bone to low-grade, chronic inflammation. Aggressive lesions such as neoplasia are more likely to produce an irregular, lytic lesion.

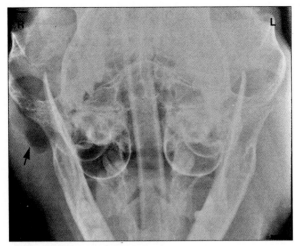

Figure 250

169 The radiograph shows a poorly marginated soft tissue swelling in the retropharynx which impinges on the nasopharynx (*Figure 251*, arrow). No bone lesion is visible.

An equine clinician faced with a swelling in this region in a horse would immediately suspect lymph node enlargement because strangles usually affects these nodes. However, it is less common to see radiographic evidence of retropharyngeal lymph node enlargement in a cat. Potential causes include metastasis from oral neoplasm, lymphoma and systemic infection. In this case, aspirate cytology of the swelling indicated lymphoma.

Figure 251

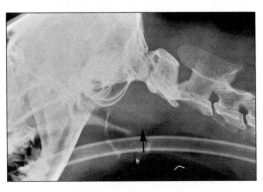

170 Three signs of death (*Figure 252*):
- Subcutaneous (S), intravascular (I) and intraperitoneal (P) gas.
- Absence of air in the lung.
- Overriding of the bones of the calvaria (arrow).

162

Gas is visible within the chambers of the heart and great vessels. As noted in a previous case, intrafoetal gas is a reliable sign of death. This case also provides an example of overriding of the bones of the calvaria (Spalding's sign) which occurs when the brain shrinks after death. (Farrow *et al.*, 1976.)

Figure 252

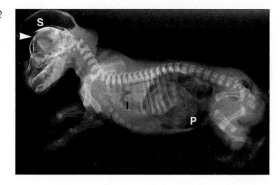

171 (a) There is enlargement and thinning of the calvaria and an open frontoparietal (bregmatic) fontanelle.
(b) The survey radiographic signs support a diagnosis of hydrocephalus.
(c) There are *four* imaging techniques that could be used to confirm hydrocephalus:
  ● Computed X-ray tomography.
  ● Magnetic resonance imaging.
  ● Pneumoventriculography (Barber *et al.*, 1987).
  ● Ultrasonography (Hudson *et al.*, 1990).
However, computed X-ray tomography and magnetic resonance imaging are not widely available.

The pneumoventriculogram in this case (rostrocaudal view, *Figure 253*) confirmed the presence of grossly enlarged lateral ventricles (arrows) compatible with hydrocephalus. An example of an ultrasound scan of a young dog with hydrocephalus is also shown (transverse view, *Figure 254*). The lateral ventricles are symmetrically enlarged (arrows).

Figure 253

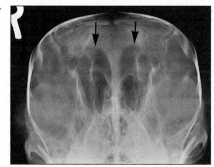

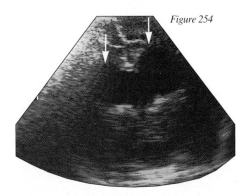

Figure 254

172 The ultrasound scan shows the lens displaced caudally and laterally, i.e. there is lens luxation.

When the cornea or anterior chamber is opaque, ultrasonography represents a useful means of evaluating the internal structures of the globe. A variety of other lesions including luxated lens, foreign body, ocular mass lesions and retinal detachments may be identified using ultrasonography (Dziezyc *et al.*, 1987).

173 A chicken furculum ('wishbone') is lodged in the proximal oesophagus, with its branches in the nasopharynx and its tip ventral to the third cervical vertebra. A few small gas lucencies in the retropharyngeal area indicate probable mucosal perforation.

The soft palate was elevated with long forceps and the bone withdrawn through the mouth. Although the oesophagus was bruised and swollen, perforation was not confirmed endoscopically.

V-shaped avian bones, such as the furculum and mandible, commonly lodge in the pharynx (Rendano *et al.*, 1988).

174 (a) There is a rounded soft tissue structure within the nasopharynx, displacing the soft palate slightly ventrally. The acute angle formed by air between the lesion and the nasopharyngeal wall indicates that it is intraluminal.
(b) An intraluminal mass in this location could be caused by nasopharyngeal polyp or foreign body.

Nasopharyngeal polyp was confirmed at surgery and was resected (Parker and Binnington, 1985).

175 This is a magnetic resonance image (MRI). Briefly, this type of image is produced by collecting radio-frequency signals from tissue placed in a strong magnetic field. The signals received depend on chemical properties of the tissue such as proton density. Using sophisticated computers it is possible to reconstruct the radio-frequency data collected from tissues into an image representing a section through the body.

The image in *Figure 193* shows the brain tissue as light grey and cerebrospinal fluid in the ventricular system as black. (The slight asymmetry of the lateral ventricles is not significant.) Cortical bone of the skull is also black and surrounding muscles are dark grey. The white layer around the ventral aspect of the head is subcutaneous fat (Kraft *et al.*, 1989).

176 (a) A highly attenuating, non-homogeneous mass (M) is visible in *Figure 255,* adjacent to the left parietal cortex. This is associated with a shift of the lateral ventricles (arrow) to the right and mild diffuse thickening of the left parietal bone (arrowheads).

(b) Meningeal or superficial cerebral mass; the parietal bone thickening is typical of meningioma (LeCouteur *et al.*, 1983).

This tumour was removed surgically. The histological diagnosis was meningioma.

Figure 255

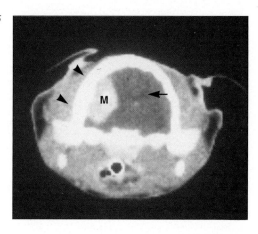

177 (a) There are four foci of increased tracer uptake in the cervical region, extending caudally to the thoracic inlet. Each of these foci represents a site of hyperactive thyroid tissue. Histological examination of such tissue usually indicates adenomatous hyperplasia. Thyroid carcinoma is uncommon in cats.

(b) The likelihood of successfully removing each of these lesions is small because they may be very small and located deep in the caudal cervical tissues, making them difficult to find at surgery. Hence this cat is a better candidate for ^{131}I treatment or long-term medical management than thyroidectomy.

Thyroid scintigraphy often reveals caudal cervical or cranial thoracic thyroid tissue which is difficult to identify by other means (Kintzer and Peterson, 1991).

REFERENCES

Ackerman, N. (1987) Radiographic aspects of heartworm disease. *Semin. Vet. Med. Surg.*, **2**, 15–27.

Ackerman, N. and Spencer, C.P. (1982) Radiologic aspects of mycotic diseases. *Vet. Clin. North Am: Small Anim. Pract.*, **12**, 175–191.

Ackerman, N. and Spencer, C.P. (1985) Radiographic diagnosis. *Vet. Radiol.*, **26**, 10–11.

Allen, G. (1986) Radiographic signs of joint disease. In: Thrall, D.E. (Ed.) *Textbook of Veterinary Diagnostic Radiology*. Philadelphia, WB Saunders Co, pp. 121–137.

Aron, D.N. (1988) Management of open musculoskeletal injuries. *Semin. Vet. Med. Surg.*, **3**, 290–301.

Barber, D.L. Oliver, J.E. and Mayhew, I.G. (1987) Neuroradiography. In: Oliver, J.E., Hoelein, B.F. and Mayhew, I.G. (Eds) *Veterinary Neurology*. Philadelphia, WB Saunders Co, pp. 65–110.

Barrett, R.B. and Kneller, S.K. (1972) Feline kidney mensuration. *Acta. Radiol. Suppl.*, **319**, 279–280.

Berg, R.J. and Wingfield, W. (1984) Pericardial effusion in the dog: a review of 42 cases. *J. Am. Anim. Hosp. Assoc.*, **20**, 721–730.

Biery, D.N. (1986) The large bowel. In: Thrall, D.E. (Ed.) *Textbook of Veterinary Diagnostic Radiology*. Philadelphia, WB Saunders Co, pp. 511–521.

Biller, D.S. and Myer, C.W. (1987) Case examples demonstrating the utility of obtaining both right and left lateral thoracic radiographs. *J. Am. Anim. Hosp. Assoc.*, **23**, 381–386.

Bohning, R.H., Suter, P.F., Hohn, R.B. and Marshall, J. (1970) Clinical and radiologic survey of canine panosteitis. *J. Am. Vet. Med. Assoc.*, **156**, 870–883.

Bonagura, J.D., O'Grady, M.R. and Herring, D.S. (1985) Echocardiography. Principles of interpretation. *Vet. Clin. North Am: Small Anim. Pract.*, **15**, 1177–1194.

Bostock, D. and White, R.A.S. (1987) Classification and behaviour after surgery of canine 'epulides'. *J. Comp. Pathol.*, **97**, 197–206.

Brearley, M.J., Thatcher, C. and Cooper, J.E. (1986) Three cases of transitional cell carcinoma in the cat and a review of the literature. *Vet. Rec.*, **118**, 91–94.

Bright, R.M., Sackman, J.E., DeNovo, C. and Toal, R. (1990) Hiatal hernia in the dog and cat: a retrospective study of 16 cases. *J. Small Anim. Pract.*, **31**, 244–250.

Brinker, W.O., Piermattei, D.L. and Flo, G.L. (1990) *Handbook of Small Animal Orthopedics and Fracture Treatment*, 2nd edn. Philadelphia, WB Saunders Co, pp. 3–5 and 250–252.

Burk, R.L., Corley, E.A. and Corwin, L.A. (1978) The radiographic appearance of pulmonary histoplasmosis in the dog and cat: a review of 37 case histories. *J. Am. Vet. Radiol. Soc.*, **19**, 2–6.

Calvert, C.A. and Brown, J. (1986) Use of M–mode echocardiography in the diagnosis of congestive cardiomyopathy in Doberman Pinschers. *J. Am. Vet. Med. Assoc.*, **189**, 293–297.

Calvert, C.A., Chapman, W.L. and Toal, R.L. (1982) Congestive cardiomyopathy in Doberman Pinscher dogs. *J. Am. Vet. Med. Assoc.*, **181**, 598–602.

Christie, B.A. (1973) Vesicoureteral reflux in dogs. *J. Am. Vet. Med. Assoc.*, **162**, 772–776.

Dallman, M.J. and Sanders, G.K. (1986) Primary spinal cord lymphosarcoma in a dog. *J. Am. Vet. Med. Assoc.* **189**, 1348–1349.

Dallman, M.J., McClure, R.C. and Brown, E.M. (1988) Histochemical study of normal and collapsed tracheas in dogs. *Am. J. Vet. Res.*, **49**, 2117–2125.

Daly, W.R. (1978) Femoral head and neck fractures in the dog and cat: a review of 115 cases. *Vet. Surg.*, **7**, 29–38.

Davies, J.V. and Read, H.M. (1990) Urethral tumours in dogs. *J. Small Anim. Pract.*, **31**, 131–136.

Dobbie, G.R., Darke, P.G.G. and Head, K.W. (1986) Intrabronchial foreign bodies in dogs. *J. Small Anim. Pract.*, **27**, 227–238.

Dziezyc, J., Hager, D.A. and Millichamp, N.J. (1987) Two-dimensional real-time ocular ultrasonography in the diagnosis of ocular lesions in dogs. *J. Am. Anim. Hosp. Assoc.*, **23**, 501–508.

Edwards, D.F., Bauer, M.S., Walker, M.A., Pardo, A.D., McCracken, M.D. and Walker, T.L. (1990) Pancreatic masses in seven dogs following acute pancreatitis. *J. Am. Anim. Hosp. Assoc.*, **26**, 189–198.

Ellison, G.W. (1980) Vascular ring anomalies in the dog and cat. *Compend. Contin. Educ. Pract. Vet.*, **2**, 693–703.

Evans, S.M. (1987) The radiographic appearance of primary liver neoplasia in dogs. *Vet. Radiol.*, **28**, 192–196.

Evans, S.J. and Biery, D.N. (1980) Congenital peritoneopericardial diaphragmatic hernia in the dog and cat: a literature review and 17 additional cases. *Vet. Radiol.*, **21**, 108–116.

Farrow, C.S (1982) Stress radiography. Applications in small animal practice. *J. Am. Vet. Med. Assoc.*, **181**, 777–784.

Farrow, C.S., Morgan, J.P. and Story, E.C. (1976) Late term fetal death in the dog: early radiographic diagnosis. *J. Am. Vet. Radiol. Soc.*, **17**, 11–17.

Feeney, D.A. (1977) Effects of dose on excretory urography. (abstract) *J. Am. Vet. Radiol. Soc.*, **18**, 34–35.

Feeney, D.A. and Johnston, G.R. (1986) The uterus. In: Thrall, D.E. (Ed.) *Textbook of Veterinary Diagnostic Radiology*. Philadelphia, WB Saunders Co, pp. 459–466.

Feeney, D.A., Johnston, G.R. Klausner, J.S., Perman, V., Leininger, J.R. and Tomlinson, M.J. (1987) Canine prostatic disease – comparison of ultrasonographic appearance with morphologic and microbiologic findings: 30 cases (1981–1985). *J. Am. Vet. Med. Assoc.*, **190**, 1018–1034.

Felts, J.F., Fox, P.R and Burk, R.L. (1984) Thread and sewing needles as gastrointestinal foreign bodies in the dog and cat: a review of 64 cases. *J. Am. Vet. Med. Assoc.*, **184**, 56–59.

Fingland, R.B., Bonagura, J.D. and Myer, C.W. (1986) Pulmonic stenosis in the dog: 29 cases (1975–1984). *J. Am. Vet. Med. Assoc.*, **189**, 218–226.

Flo, G.L., Stickle, R.L. and Dunstan, R.W. (1987) Synovial chondrometaplasia in five dogs. *J. Am. Vet. Med. Assoc.*, **191**,1417–1422.

Fossum, T.W., Evering, W.N., Miller, M.W., Forrester, S.D., Palmer, D.R. and Hodges, C.C. (1992) Severe bilateral fibrosing pleuritis associated with chronic chylothorax in five cats and two dogs. *J. Am. Vet. Med. Assoc.*, **201**, 317–324.

Gibbons, G. and Murtaugh, R.J. (1990) Cecal smooth muscle neoplasia in the dog: report of 11 cases and literature review. *J. Am. Anim. Hosp. Assoc.*, **25**, 191–197.

Gibbs, C. and Pearson, H. (1973) The radiological diagnosis of gastrointestinal obstruction in the dog. *J. Small Anim. Pract.*, **14**, 61–82.

Gibbs, C. and Pearson, H. (1986) Localized tumours of the canine small intestine: a report of twenty cases. *J. Small Anim. Pract.*, **27**, 507–519.

Gibbs, C., Denny, H.R. and Kelly, D.F. (1984) The radiological features of osteosarcoma of the appendicular skeleton in dogs, a review of 74 cases. *J. Small Anim. Pract.*, **25**, 177–192.

Gilmore, D.R. (1983) Intraspinal tumors in the dog. *Compend. Contin. Educ. Pract. Vet.*, **5**, 55–64.

Grondalen, J. (1976) Metaphyseal osteopathy (hypertrophic osteodystrophy) in growing dogs. A clinical study. *J. Small Anim. Pract.*, **17**, 721–735.

Harvey, C.E., Biery, D.N., Morello, J. and O'Brien, J.A. (1979) Chronic nasal disease in the dog: its radiographic diagnosis. *J. Am. Vet. Radiol. Soc.*, **20**, 91–98.

167

Hudson, J.A., Simpson, S.T., Buxton, D.F., Cartee, R.E. and Steiss, J.E. (1990) Ultrasonographic diagnosis of canine hydrocephalus. *Vet. Radiol.* **31**, 50–58.

Johnson, C.A., Armstrong, P.J. and Hauptman, J.G. (1987) Congenital portosystemic shunts in dogs: 46 cases (1979–1986). *J. Am. Vet. Med. Assoc.*, **191**, 1478–1483.

Johnston, D.E. and Summers, B.A. (1971) Osteomyelitis of the lumbar vertebrae in the dog caused by grass-seed foreign bodies. *Aust. Vet. J.*, **47**, 289–294.

Kerr, D.V. and Kirker-Head, C. (1989) What is your diagnosis? *J. Am. Vet. Med. Assoc.*, **195**, 383–384.

Kintzer, P.P. and Peterson, M.E. (1991) Thyroid scintigraphy in small animals. *Semin. Vet. Med. Surg.*, **6**, 131–139.

Konde, L.J. and Spaulding, K. (1991) Sonographic evaluation of the mediastinum in small animals. *Vet. Radiol.*, **32**, 178–184.

Kraft, S.L., Gavin, P.R., Wendling, L.R. and Reddy, V.K. (1989) Canine brain anatomy on magnetic resonance images. *Vet. Radiol.*, **30**, 147–158.

Kramers, P., Flückiger M.A., Rahn, B.A. and Cordey, J. (1988) Osteopetrosis in cats. *J. Small Anim. Pract.*, **29**, 153–164.

Kremkau, K.W. and Taylor, K.J.W. (1986) Artifacts in ultrasound imaging. *J. Ultrasound Med.*, **5**, 227–237.

Lamb, C.R. (1991a) The principles and practice of bone scintigraphy in small animals. *Semin. Vet. Med. Surg.*, **6**, 140–153.

Lamb, C.R. (1991b) Ultrasonography of the liver and biliary tract. In: Kaplan, P.M. (Ed.) *Problems in Veterinary Medicine, Volume 3, Ultrasound*. Philadelphia, Lippincott, pp. 555–573.

Lamb, C.R., Hartzband, L.E., Tidwell, A.S. and Pearson, S.H. (1991a) Ultrasonographic findings in hepatic and splenic lymphosarcoma in dogs and cats. *Vet. Radiol.*, **32**, 117–120.

Lamb, C.R., Kleine, L.J. and McMillan, M.C. (1991b) Diagnosis of calcification on abdominal radiographs. *Vet. Radiol.*, **32**, 211–220.

LeCouteur, R.A., Fike, J.R., Cann, C.E., Turrel, J.M., Thompson, J.E. and Biggart, J.F. (1983) X-ray computed tomography of brain tumors in cats. *J. Am. Vet. Med. Assoc.*, **183**, 301–305.

Lee, R. (1974) Legg-Perthes disease in the dog: the histological and associated radiological changes. *J. Am. Vet. Radiol. Soc.*, **15**, 24–27.

Ling, G.V., Morgan, J.P. and Pool, R.R. (1974) Primary bone tumors in the dog: a combined clinical, radiographic, and histologic approach to early diagnosis. *J. Am. Vet. Med. Assoc.*, **165**, 55–67.

Lord, P.F. (1975) Neurogenic pulmonary edema in the dog. *J. Am. Anim. Hosp. Assoc.*, **11**, 778–783.

Lord, P.F., Carb, A., Halliwell, W.H. and Prueter, J.C. (1982) Emphysematous hepatic abscess associated with trauma, necrotic hepatic nodular hyperplasia and adenoma in a dog: a case history report. *Vet. Radiol.*, **23**, 46–49.

Lord, P.F. and Gomez, J.A. (1985) Lung lobe collapse. Pathophysiology and radiologic signficance. *Vet. Radiol.*, **26**, 187–195.

Luis Fuentes, V. (1992) Feline heart disease: an update. *J. Small Anim. Pract.*, **33**, 130–137.

Lust, G., Rendano, V.T. and Summers, B.A. (1985) Canine hip dysplasia: concepts and diagnosis. *J. Am. Vet. Med. Assoc.*, **187**, 638–640.

Marks, S.L., Bellak, J.R. and Wells, M. (1991) Resolution of quadriparesis caused by cervical tumoral calcinosis in a dog. *J. Am. Anim. Hosp. Assoc.*, **27**, 72–76.

Mason, L.K., Stone, E.A., Biery, D.N., Robertson, I. and Thrall, D.E. (1990) Surgery of ectopic ureters: pre- and postoperative radiographic morphology. *J. Am. Anim. Hosp. Assoc.*, **26**, 73–79.

Mayrhofer, E. (1985) Radiological diagnosis of stone kernels in the small intestine in dogs. *Wein Tierärztl. Mschr.*, **72**, 151–154.

McKee, W.M. (1990) Spinal trauma in dogs and cats: a review of 51 cases. *Vet. Rec.,* **126**, 285–289.

McNeel, S.V. (1986) The small bowel. In: Thrall, D.E. (Ed.) *Textbook of Veterinary Diagnostic Radiology*. Philadelphia, WB Saunders Co, pp. 493–510.

Mee, A.P., Webber, D.M., May, C., Bennett, D., Sharpe, P.T. and Anderson, D.C. (1992) Detection of canine distemper virus in bone cells in the metaphyses of distemper–infected dogs. *J. Bone Min. Res.,* **7**, 829–834.

Middleton, W.D. and Melson, G.L. (1988) Diaphragmatic discontinuity associated with perihepatic ascites: a sonographic refractive artifact. *Am. J. Roentgenol.,***151**, 709–711.

Miller, J.B. and Sande, R.D. (1980) Osseous metaplasia in the renal pelvis of a dog with hydronephrosis. *Vet. Radiol.,* **21**, 146–148.

Mitten, R.W. (1974) Vertebral osteomyelitis in the dog due to Nocardia-like organisms. *J. Small Anim. Pract.,* **15**, 563–570.

Mitten, R.W. (1982) Radiology of mediastinal diseases. *Vet. Clin. North Am: Small Anim. Pract.,* **12**, 193–211.

Morgan, J.P. (1981) The upper gastrointestinal examination in the cat: normal radiographic appearance using positive contrast medium. *Vet. Radiol.,* **22**, 159–169.

Morgan, J.P. and Rosenblatt, L. (1987) Canine hip dysplasia: significance of pelvic and sacral attachment. *Calif. Vet..* **41**, 12–16.

Morgan, J.P., Ackerman, N., Bailey, C.S. and Pool, R.R.(1980) Vertebral tumors in the dog: a clinical, radiologic, and pathologic study of 61 primary and secondary lesions. *Vet. Radiol.,* **21**, 197–212.

Moroff, S.D., Brown, B.A., Matthiesen, D.T. and Scott, R.C. (1991) Infiltrative urethral disease in female dogs: 41 cases (1980–1987). *J. Am. Vet. Med. Assoc.,* **199**, 247–251.

Moulton, J.E. (1990) *Tumors in Domestic Animals*, 3rd edn. Berkeley, University of California Press.

Mucci, B. and Stenhouse, G. (1985) Soft tissue radiography for wooden foreign bodies – a worthwhile exercise. *Injury,* **16**, 402–404.

Myer, C.W. and Burk, J.K. (1973) Bronchiectasis in the dog: its radiographic appearance. *J. Am. Vet. Radiol. Soc.,* **14**, 3–12.

Nunamaker, D.M., Rhinelander, F.W. and Heppenstall, R.B. (1985) Delayed union, nonunion, malunion. In: Newton, C.D. and Nunamaker, D.M. (Eds) *Textbook of Small Animal Orthopedics*. Philadelphia, JB Lippincott Co, pp. 511–518.

Nyland, T.G. and Kantrowitz, B.M. (1986) Ultrasound in the diagnosis and staging of abdominal neoplasia. In: Gorman, N.T. (Ed.) *Contemporary Issues in Small Animal Practice, Volume 6, Oncology*. New York, Churchill Livingstone, pp. 1–24.

Olsson, S-E. (1983) The early diagnosis of fragmented coronoid process and osteochondrosis dissecans of the canine elbow joint. *J. Am. Anim. Hosp. Assoc.,* **19**, 616–626.

Padrid, P.A., Hornof, W.J., Kurpershoek, C.J. and Cross, C.E (1990) Canine chronic bronchitis. A pathophysiological evaluation of 18 cases. *J. Vet. Intern. Med.,* **4**, 172–180.

Parker, N.R. and Binnington, A.G. (1985) Nasopharyngeal polyps in cats: three case reports and a review of the literature. *J. Am. Anim. Hosp. Assoc.,* **21**, 473–478.

Penninck, D.G., Nyland, T.G., Kerr, L.Y. and Fisher, P.E. (1990) Ultrasonographic evaluation of gastrointestinal diseases in small animals. *Vet. Radiol.,* **31**, 134–141.

Phillips, L., Hager, D., Parker, R. and Yanik, D. (1986) Osteosarcoma with a pathological fracture in a six–month old dog. *Vet. Radiol.,* **27**, 18–19.

Poulos, P.W. (1982) Canine osteochondrosis. *Vet. Clin. North Am: Small Anim. Pract.,* **12**, 313–328.

Prymak, C., McKee, L.J., Goldschmidt, M.H. and Glickman, L.T. (1988) Epidemiologic, clinical, pathologic, and prognostic characteristics of splenic hemangiosarcoma and splenic hematoma in dogs: 217 cases (1985). *J. Am. Vet. Med. Assoc.*, **193**, 706–712.

Quigley, P.J. and Leedale, A.H. (1983) Tumors involving bone in the domestic cat: a review of fifty-eight cases. *Vet. Pathol.*, **20**, 670–686.

Reiderson, T.H., Metz, A.L. and Hardy, R.M. (1988) Thoracic vertebral osteochondroma in a cat. *J. Am. Vet. Med. Assoc.*, 192, 1102–1104.

Rendano, V. (1979) Positive contrast peritoneography: an aid in radiographic diagnosis of diaphragmatic hernia. *J. Am. Vet. Radiol. Soc.*, **20**, 67–73.

Rendano, V., Zimmer, J.F., Wallach, M.S. Jacobson, R. and Pudalov, I. (1988) Impaction of the pharynx, larynx and esophagus by avian bones in the dog and cat. *Vet. Radiol.*, **29**, 213–216.

Riser, W.H., Parkes, L.J. and Shirer, J.F. (1967) Canine craniomandibular osteopathy. *J. Am. Vet. Radiol. Soc.*, **8**, 23–31.

Root, C.R. and Lord, P.F. (1971) Radiolucent gastrointestinal foreign bodies in cats and dogs. *J. Am. Vet. Radiol. Soc.*, **12**, 45–53.

Root, C.R. and Scott, R.C. (1971) Emphysematous cystitis and other radiographic manifestations of diabetes mellitus in dogs and cats. *J. Am. Vet. Med. Assoc.*, **158**, 721–728.

Rush, J.E., Keene, B.W. and Fox, P.R. (1990) Pericardial disease in the cat: a retrospective evaluation of 66 cases. *J. Am. Anim. Hosp. Assoc.*, **26**, 39–46.

Russel, R.G. and Walker, M. (1983) Metastatic and invasive tumors of bone in dogs and cats. *Vet. Clin. North Am: Small Anim. Pract.*, **13**, 163–179.

Schmidt, M. and Wolvecamp, P. (1991) Radiographic findings in ten dogs with thoracic actinomycosis. *Vet. Radiol.*, **32**, 301–306.

Schmidt, S. and Suter, P.F. (1980) Angiography of the hepatic and portal venous system in the dog and cat: an investigative method. *Vet. Radiol.*, **21**, 57–77.

Scott, D.W. and Buerger, R.G. (1988) Idiopathic calcinosis circumscripta in the dog: a retrospective analysis of 130 cases. *J. Am. Anim. Hosp. Assoc.*, **24**, 651–658.

Seim, H.B. and Withrow, S.J. (1982) Pathophysiology and diagnosis of caudal cervical spondylomyelopathy with emphasis on the Doberman Pinscher. *J. Am. Anim. Hosp. Assoc.*, **18**, 241–251.

Selcer, B.A. (1982) Urinary tract trauma associated with pelvic trauma. *J. Am. Anim. Hosp. Assoc.*, **18**, 785–793.

Selcer, R.R., Bubb, W.J. and Waller, T.L. (1991) Management of vertebral column fractures in dogs and cats: 211 cases (1977–1985). *J. Am. Vet. Med. Assoc.*, **198**, 1965–1968.

Sevelius E., Tidholm A. and Thoren–Tolling K. (1990) Pyometra in the dog. *J. Am. Anim. Hosp. Assoc.*, **26**, 33–38.

Shields-Henney, L.H. and Gambardella, P.C. (1989) Premature closure of the ulnar physis in the dog: a retrospective clinical study. *J. Am. Anim. Hosp. Assoc.*, **25**, 573–581.

Slocum, B. and Devine, T.M. (1990) Dorsal acetabular rim radiographic view for evaluation of the canine hip. *J. Am. Anim. Hosp. Assoc.*, **26**, 289–296.

Snyder, P.S., Sato, T. and Atkins, C.E. (1990) The utility of thoracic radiographic measurement for the detection of cardiomegaly in cats with pleural effusion. *Vet. Radiol.,* **31**, 89–91.

Spackman, C.J.A., Caywood, D.D., Johnston, G.R. and Feeney, D.A. (1984) Granulomas of the ovarian and uterine stumps: a case report. *J. Am. Anim. Hosp. Assoc.*, **20**, 449–453.

Stowater, J.L. and Lamb, C.R. (1989) Ultrasonography of non-cardiac thoracic diseases in small animals. *J. Am. Vet. Med. Assoc.*, **195**, 514–520.

Sullivan, M., Lee, R., Jakovljevic, S. and Sharp, N.J.H. (1986) The radiological features of aspergillosis of the nasal cavity and frontal sinuses of the dog. *J. Small Anim. Pract.*, **27**, 167–180.

Sullivan, M., Lee, R., Skae, C.A. (1987) The radiological features of sixty cases of intranasal neoplasia in the dog. *J. Small Anim. Pract.*, **28**, 575–586.

Thomas, W.P., Reed, J.R. and Gomez, J.A. (1984) Diagnostic pneumopericardiography in dogs with spontaneous pericardial effusion. *Vet. Radiol.*, **25**, 2–16.

Thrall, D.E. (1981) Radiographic aspects of prostatic diseases in the dog. *Compend. Contin. Educ. Pract. Vet.*, **3**, 718–724.

Thrall, D.E. (1986) Opacity and density. *Vet. Radiol.*, **27**, 162–163.

Ticer, J.W. (1984) *Radiographic Technique in Veterinary Practice,* 2nd edn. Philadelphia, WB Saunders Co, p. 107.

van Bree, H. and Sackx, A. (1987) Evaluation of radiographic liver size in twenty-seven normal deep-chested dogs. *J. Small Anim. Pract.*, **28**, 693–703.

van Bree, H., van Ryssen, B. and Desmidt, M. (1992) Osteochondrosis lesions of the canine shoulder: correlation of positive contrast arthrography and arthroscopy. *Vet. Radiol.*, **33**, 342–347.

van den Broek, A.H.M. and Darke, P.G.G. (1987) Cardiac measurements on thoracic radiographs of cats. *J. Small Anim. Pract.*, **28**, 125–135.

Vessal, K., Montali, R.J., Larson, S.M., Chaffee, V. and James. A.E. (1975) Evaluation of barium and gastrografin as contrast media for the diagnosis of esophageal ruptures or perforations. *Am. J. Roentgenol.*, **123**, 307–319.

Walter, P.A,. Johnston, G.R., Feeney, D.A. and O'Brien, T.D. (1988) Applications of ultrasonography in the diagnosis of parenchymal kidney disease in cats: 24 cases (1981–1986). *J. Am. Vet. Med. Assoc.*, **192**, 92–98.

Waters, D.J., Caywood, D.D., Hayden, D.W. and Klausner, J.S. (1988) Metastatic pattern in dogs with splenic haemangiosarcoma: clinical implications. *J. Small Anim. Pract.*, **29**, 805–814.

Wegener, M., Borsch, G., Schneider, J., Wedmann, B., Winter, R. and Zacharias, J. (1987) Gallbladder wall thickening: a frequent finding in various non-biliary disorders – a prospective ultrasonographic study. *J. Clin. Ultrasound*, **15**, 307–312.

White, R.A.S. and Herrtage, M.E. (1986) Bladder retroflexion in the dog. *J. Small Anim. Pract.*, **27**, 735–746.

White, R.A.S., Herrtage, M.E. and Dennis, R. (1987) The diagnosis and management of paraprostatic and prostatic retention cysts in the dog. *J. Small Anim. Pract.*, **28**, 551–574.

Woodard, J.C. (1982) Canine hypertrophic osteodystrophy, a study of the spontaneous disease in littermates. *Vet. Pathol.*, **19**, 337–354.

INDEX

Numbers refer to Question and Answer numbers.

Abdomen
    abdominal wall mass 60
    abscess 86
    pseudomass 87
Abrasion injuries 126
Abscesses
    abdominal 86
    kidney 66
    liver 57, 78, 102
    lung 49
    mediastinal 48
    tooth root 140
Acetabular rim, dorsal 130
Air trapping 50
Anaemia, chronic 52
Anconeal process, ununited 110, 133
Aortic lesions 48
Artefacts 33, 105, 108
Arthritis, bacterial 125, 132
Arthrography 153
Articular fractures 133
Ascariasis 83
Ascites 101, 103
Aspergillosis 166
Atresia coli 63
Atrium
    enlarged 29, 30, 40
    ruptured left 45
Avulsion fractures 133

Barbiturates 52
Bladder
    carcinoma 85, 88
    herniation 74
    mis-shapen 74
    retroflexion 89
Blastomycosis 49
Blurring 5, 6
Bone
    scintigraphy 141,
    tumours 129, 140, 149, 151, 160, 162
    see also Fractures; Osteomyelits
Bronchiectasis 37
Bronchitis
    chronic 19
    localised 47
Bronchopneumonia 10, 25, 26, 27, 33
Bronchoscopy 47

Bronchus, obstructed 47
Bucky factor 8
Bullae, lung 49, 50

Calcinosis circumscripta (tumoral calcinosis)
    133, 147
Calcification 23, 52, 57, 68, 75, 133, 153
Calculus, urinary 108
Carcinoma
    bile duct 86
    bladder 85, 88
    intestine 62, 95, 97, 107
    liver 56, 102
    mammary 123
    nail-bed 161
    pancreatic 86
    prostatic 73, 123, 141
    squamous cell 140
    sweat-gland 161
    thyroid 31, 41, 123
    urethral 72
    see also Tumours
Carcinomatosis 36
Cardiac failure 13, 20
Cardiomegaly 17, 26, 29, 40
Cardiomyopathy, hypertrophic 13, 27, 30, 45
Carpal arthrosis 144
Cartilage flap 133, 153
Chemodectoma 31, 41, 45, 48
Cholangiohepatitis, ascending 57
Cholecystitis 103
    emphysematous 78, 82
Chondrometaplasia, synovial 147
Chylothorax 20, 22
Cirrhosis 101, 103
Coagulopathy 45
Computed X-ray tomography 176
Congestive heart failure 45, 103
Contrast radiography 58, 63, 72, 74, 83, 85,
    86, 88, 89, 91, 93–97, 99, 100, 134–138,
    153, 157, 158, 162
Cough 10, 19, 34, 37, 40
Coxofemoral joint
    calcification 147
    luxation 110, 142
Cystic mucinous hyperplasia 103
Cystitis
    emphysematous 82

Cystitis *continued*
    polypoid 70
    ulcerated 85
Cystogram 70
    negative-contrast 98
Cysts
    intraprostatic 68, 93
    kidney 66
    liver 102
    lung 49
    mediastinal 48
    paraprostatic 60, 68, 90, 93
    pericardial 45

Degenerative joint disease 125, 131, 144
Dental eruption, complete 164
Dental formulae 163
Diabetes mellitus 82, 90
Diaphragm
    caudal displacement 46
    ruptured 21, 39
Dirofilaria immitis infection (heartworm
    disease) 44
Duodenum, plication 94
Dysphagia 15
Dyspnoea 22, 25, 28
Dystocia 170

Elbow arthrosis 131
Electrocution 35
Embolism, pulmonary 25, 47, 50
Emphysema 50, 118
End-on pulmonary vessels 32
Endocardiosis 29
Enteritis 58, 86
Enthesopathy 119
Epilepsy 35
Epulis 140
Exostosis, ossifying cartilagenous 162
Exposure time 6, 7

Fat deposits 31
Fat necrosis, mesenteric 90
Femur
    fractures 114
    ischaemic necrosis of head
        (Legg–Calvé–Perthes disease) 154
Fibrosarcoma 140
Fibular fracture 145
Foetus, dead 81, 170
Foreign bodies
    duodenal 94

Foreign bodies *continued*
    inhaled 25, 47
    linear 94
    migrating 158, 159
    nasopharynx 165
    osteomyelitis 129
    small intestinal obstruction 77
    wooden 155
Fractures
    callus 162
    fibular 145
    malunion 146, 152
    metacarpal 128
    pathological 149
    phalangeal 127
    physeal 124
    radial 146
    Salter–Harris
    type ii 145
    type iv 124
    tibial 145
    vertebrae, compression 143

Gingival lesions, inflammatory 140
Glomerulonephritis 66
Granulomas 31, 49
Gravel sign 62
Growth plates 109

Haemangiosarcoma 123, 150
    atrial 41, 45
    extradural 158
    mediastinal 48
    splenic 36, 54
Haematoma
    extradural 158
    liver 102
    mediastinal 9, 31, 48
Haematuria 73, 74, 76, 88, 93
Haemoptysis 25
Haemorrhage
    intraocular 172
    localised 47
    pulmonary 25, 27
    renal 65
    traumatic 20, 25
Heart
    radiographic identification 4
    size 12
    see Cardiomegaly; Cardiomyopathy;
    Congestive heart failure; Cardiac failure
Heartworm disease 44

Hemilaminectomy 157, 158
Hepatic nodular hyperplasia 102
Hepatitis 102, 103
Hepatozoonosis 159
Hernia
    congenital peritoneopericardial
        diaphragmatic 24
    hiatal 46
    inguinal 84
    perineal 89
Hip dysplasia 116, 130
Histoplasmosis 43, 52
Humeroradial subluxation 124
Humeroulnar subluxation 124, 146
Hydrocephalus 171
Hydronephrosis 65, 66, 74, 106
Hydroureter 74
Hyperthyroidism 27, 177
Hypoalbuminaemia 103
Hypoglycaemia 35
Hypovolaemia 28, 36, 50

Infarct, pulmonary 47
Inguinal mass 84
Intervertebral disc
    disc space narrowing 117
    prolapse 157, 158
Intestine
    atresia 63
    intussusception 64
Intestinal obstruction
    complete 61, 77
    partial 62, 94, 97
    neoplasm 62, 95, 97, 107
Intrameniscal calcification 133
Intrathoracic mass 10
Intussusception 64

Jejunum
    lymphoma 79
    neoplasm 62
Joints
    arthrosis 125, 131, 144
    calcified lesions 133
    see also Degenerative joint disease;
    Arthritis, bacterial; Osteochondrosis;
    Arthrography

Kidneys
    abscess 66
    asymmetrical 66
    bilaterally enlarged 65
    calcification 75
    cyst 66

Kidneys continued
    end-stage disease 75
    failure 23
    hydronephrosis 65, 66, 74, 106
    hypertrophy 66
    hypoplasia 66
    lymphoma 65, 66, 106
    normal length 53
    polycystic 65, 100
    pyelonephritis 66, 106
    radiographic identification 4
    tumour 76

Lead poisoning 122
Legg-Calvé-Perthes disease 154
Leiomyoma 72
Leptospirosis 65
Ligaments, ruptured cruciate 120
Ligamentum arteriosum, ligation and division
    14
Light fogging 111
Linear foreign body 94
Lipoma, extradural 158
Liver
    abscess 57, 78, 102
    calcification 57
    carcinoma 56, 102
    cirrhosis 101, 103
    haematoma 102
    hypoechoic lesions 102
    lymphoma 102
    metastases 62, 102
    normal size 51
Lungs
    abscess 49
    collapse 28, 38
    hyperlucent 50
    infiltrates 25, 27, 42, 47
    lymphoma 33
    mass 10, 11
    metastases 33, 36, 49, 161
    opacity 13, 33
    tumour, primary 49
Lymph nodes
    calcification 43
    enlargement 18, 31, 42, 59, 84
    metastases 31, 59
Lymphoid hyperplasia 52
Lymphoma 9, 18, 45
    extradural 158
    intestinal 107
    jejunal 79
    kidney 65, 66, 106
    liver 102

Lymphoma *continued*
    lung 33
    mediastinal 31, 48
    retropharyngeal 169
    spleen 52, 55, 104

Magnetic resonance imaging (MRI) 175
Marie's disease 121
Medial condyle fracture 124
Mediastinum
    mass 9, 31, 46, 48
    shift 9, 10, 28, 38
Megaoesophagus 34
Meningioma 176
Mesenteric mass 60
Mesothelioma 60
Metacarpal fractures 128
Metastases
    bone 123
    liver 62, 102
    lymph node 31, 59
    osseous 121
    pulmonary 33, 36, 49, 161
Metastatic calcification 23
Mirror-image artefact 105
Mitral valve lesions 29
Mycosis
    granuloma 49
    systemic 31, 45
    thoracic 42, 43
Myelography
    examples 137, 157, 158, 162
    filling defects 137
    indications 135
    injection sites 134
    lesion location 136

Nail-bed neoplasm 161
Nasal discharge 165, 166, 167, 174
Near-drowning 26
Neoplasms *see* Carcinoma; Haemangio-
    sarcoma; Lymphoma; Tumours
Nephritis 65, 106

Obstruction *see* Intestine
Oedema, pulmonary 13, 25, 26, 27, 33, 34, 40
Oesophagram 15, 16
Oesophagus
    dilated 31, 34, 46, 48
    obstruction 14, 173
    ruptured 16
Old dog lung 33
Opacity 2

Osteochondroma (ossifying cartilagenous
    exostosis) 162
Osteochondrometaplasia, synovial 133
Osteochondrosis 110, 125, 133, 153
Osteodystrophy, hypertrophic (metaphyseal
    osteopathy) 115, 122
Osteomyelitis 129, 150, 159, 162
Osteopathy
    craniomandibular 148
    hypertrophic (Marie's disease) 121
    metaphyseal 115, 122
Osteopenia 128
Osteopetrosis 139
Osteosarcoma 129, 151
Otitis media 168
Over-development 111
Over-exposure 50, 111

Pancreatic mass 60, 86
Pancreatitis 86
Panosteitis 113, 121
Paragonimus spp. infection 49
Paraplegia 28, 143, 157, 159
Patella, luxation 118
Pathological fractures 149
Pelvic attachment, asymmetrical 142
Pelvis, trauma 74, 114
Pericardial cyst 45
Pericardial fluid 41, 45
Peritoneum
    adhesions 36
    fluid 36, 63
Peritonitis, feline infectious 20, 45, 66, 106
Phalangeal fracture 127
Phenothiazine 52
Photographic density 1
Pleural fluid 20, 22, 39, 42
Pleuritis 22
Pneumocystogram 85, 88
Pneumohaemothorax 39
Pneumomediastinum 28
Pneumonia
    aspiration 34
    inhalation 27
Pneumonitis 33
Pneumopericardiogram 41
Pneumoperitoneum 78
Pneumothorax 22, 38
Pneumoventriculogram 171
Polycystic kidney disease 65, 100
Polydipsia 18, 82, 84, 90, 92, 108, 169
Polyp, nasopharyngeal 174
Polyuria 18, 82, 90, 92, 108

175

Portogram, operative mesenteric 91, 96
Portosystemic shunts, congenital 65, 96
Prostate
    benign hypertrophy 93
    calcified lesions 68
    carcinoma 73, 123, 141
    normal 67
    reflux, urethrography 69
Prostatitis, chronic 68
Prostatomegaly 73
Pseudomass 87
Pulmonic stenosis 17
Pyelonephritis 66, 106
Pyogranuloma 80
Pyometra 92
Pyothorax 20, 22

Radial fracture 146
Refraction 105
Regurgitation 14, 15, 46
Renal failure 103
Renal pelvis, osseous metaplasia 76
    see Hydronephrosis
Rhinitis, fungal 166
Rickets 122

Sacroiliac joint asymmetry 142
Scintigraphy
    bone 141
    thyroid 177
Sertoli-cell tumour 84
Shunt, portacaval 65, 96
Smoke inhalation 25, 26
Spinal cord
    injury 117
    lesions 138
    oedema 157
    see Myelography
Spindle-cell sarcoma 160
Spleen
    hypoechoic lesion 104
    lymphoma 52, 55, 104
    mass 36
    neoplasm 60
Splenomegaly 52, 55
Spondylosis deformans 62, 79
Squamous cell carcinoma 140
Stifle arthrosis 125
Stomach, displacement 21, 56
Sweat-gland carcinoma 161

Tarsal joint instability 119
Tendinopathy, calcified 133

Testicle, retained 60, 84, 90
Tetralogy of Fallot 17
Thoracocentesis 22
Thymoma 9, 31
Thyroid neoplasm 123
    ectopic 31, 41
    scintigraphy 177
Tibial fracture 145
Tissue types 3
Tooth fragments 118
Tooth root abscess 140
Trachea
    collapse 40
    displaced 48
Tumours
    bone 129, 140, 149, 151, 160, 162
    kidney 76
    leiomyoma 72
    lung 49
    meningioma 176
    primary nasal 166, 167
    Sertoli-cell 84
    see also Carcinoma; Haemangiosarcoma;
    Lymphoma

Ulnar fracture 146
Ultrasonography 21, 29, 39, 65, 79, 80,
    101–108, 172
Urachal diverticulum 85
Uraemia 45
Ureters
    normal 98
    bilateral ectopic 99
    ruptured 74
Ureterocoele 70
Urethral neoplasm 72
Urethrography 69, 72
Urinary calculus 108
Urogram, intravenous 71, 98
Urolith 70
Uterine stump lesions 80
Uterus, enlarged 92

Vaginal discharge 81
Vaginourethrogram 72
Vascular ring anomaly 14
Vascular stasis 52
Ventral mid-abdominal mass 60
Vertebrae, compression fracture 143
Vesicoureteral reflux 89

Zygomatic arch fracture 110